MICROWAVE COOKBOOK 2022

TASTY AND DELICIOUS RECIPES FOR BEGINNERS

JENNA FONDA

Table of Contents

Braised Beef and Vegetables 14
Beef Stew 15
Beef and Vegetable Hot-pot 16
Beef Curry 17
Basic Mince 18
Cottage Pie 19
Cottage Pie with Cheese 19
Mince with Oats 20
Chilli con Carne 20
Curried Mince 21
Beef Goulash 22
Beef Goulash with Boiled Potatoes 23
Butter Bean and Beef Stew with Tomatoes 23
Beef and Tomato Cake 24
Beef and Mushroom Kebabs 25
Stuffed Lamb 27
Minted Lamb Kebabs 28
Classic Lamb Kebabs 29
Middle Eastern Lamb with Fruit 30
Mock Irish Stew 31
Farmer's Wife Lamb Chops 32
Lamb Hot-pot 33

Lamb Loaf with Mint and Rosemary 34
Lamb Bredie with Tomatoes 35
Lamb Biriani 36
Ornate Biriani 37
Moussaka 38
Moussaka with Potatoes 39
Quick Moussaka 40
Lamb Mince 41
Shepherd's Pie 41
Country Liver in Red Wine 42
Liver and Bacon 43
Liver and Bacon with Apple 44
Kidneys in Red Wine with Brandy 45
Venison Steaks with Oyster Mushrooms and Blue Cheese 47
Cooking Small Pasta 48
Chinese Noodle and Mushroom Salad with Walnuts 48
Pepper Macaroni 49
Family Macaroni Cheese 50
Classic Macaroni Cheese 51
Macaroni Cheese with Stilton 52
Macaroni Cheese with Bacon 52
Macaroni Cheese with Tomatoes 52
Spaghetti Carbonara 53
Pizza-style Macaroni Cheese 54
Spaghetti Cream with Spring Onions 55
Spaghetti Bolognese 56
Spaghetti with Turkey Bolognese Sauce 57

Spaghetti with Ragu Sauce 58
Spaghetti with Butter 59
Pasta with Garlic 60
Spaghetti with Beef and Mixed Vegetable Bolognese Sauce 61
Spaghetti with Meat Sauce and Cream 62
Spaghetti with Marsala Meat Sauce 62
Pasta alla Marinara 63
Pasta Matriciana 64
Pasta with Tuna and Capers 65
Pasta Napoletana 66
Pasta Pizzaiola 67
Pasta with Peas 67
Pasta with Chicken Liver Sauce 67
Pasta with Anchovies 68
Ravioli with Sauce 68
Tortellini 69
Lasagne 70
Pizza Napoletana 71
Pizza Margherita 72
Seafood Pizza 72
Pizza Siciliana 72
Mushroom Pizza 72
Ham and Pineapple Pizza 73
Pepperoni Pizzas 73
Buttered Flaked Almonds 74
Flaked Almonds in Garlic Butter 74
Dried Chestnuts 74

Drying Herbs	75
Crisping Breadcrumbs	76
Nut Burgers	77
Nutkin Cake	78
Buckwheat	79
Bulgar	80
Bulgar with Fried Onion	81
Tabbouleh	82
Sultan's Salad	83
Couscous	84
Grits	85
Gnocchi alla Romana	86
Ham Gnocchi	87
Millet	88
Polenta	89
Grilled Polenta	90
Polenta with Pesto	90
Polenta with Sun-dried Tomato or Olive Paste	90
Quinoa	91
Romanian Polenta	92
Curried Rice	93
Cottage Cheese and Rice Casserole	94
Italian Risotto	95
Mushroom Risotto	96
Brazilian Rice	96
Spanish Rice	97
Plain Turkish Pilaf	98

Rich Turkish Pilaf 99
Thai Rice with Lemon Grass, Lime Leaves and Coconut 100
Okra with Cabbage 101
Red Cabbage with Apple 102
Red Cabbage with Wine 104
Norwegian Sour Cabbage 104
Greek-style Stewed Okra with Tomatoes 105
Greens with Tomatoes, Onions and Peanut Butter 106
Sweet-sour Creamed Beetroot 107
Beetroot in Orange 108
Scalloped Celeriac 109
Celeriac with Orange Hollandaise Sauce 110
Slimmers' Vegetable Pot 111
Slimmers' Vegetable Pot with Eggs 111
Ratatouille 112
Caramelised Parsnips 113
Parsnips with Egg and Butter Crumb Sauce 114
Broccoli with Cheese Supreme 115
Guvetch 116
Celery Cheese with Bacon 117
Artichoke Cheese with Bacon 118
Karelian Potatoes 119
Dutch Potato and Gouda Casserole with Tomatoes 120
Buttered and Fluffed Sweet Potatoes with Cream 121
Maître d'Hôtel Sweet Potatoes 122
Creamed Potatoes 122
Creamed Potatoes with Parsley 123

Creamed Potatoes with Cheese	*123*
Hungarian Potatoes with Paprika	*124*
Dauphine Potatoes	*125*
Savoyard Potatoes	*126*
Château Potatoes	*126*
Potatoes with Almond Butter Sauce	*127*
Mustard and Lime Tomatoes	*128*
Braised Cucumber	*129*
Braised Cucumber with Pernod	*129*
Marrow Espagnole	*130*
Gratin of Courgettes and Tomatoes	*131*
Courgettes with Juniper Berries	*132*
Buttered Chinese Leaves with Pernod	*133*
Chinese-style Bean Sprouts	*134*
Carrots with Orange	*135*
Braised Chicory	*136*
Braised Carrots with Lime	*137*
Fennel in Sherry	*138*
Wine-braised Leeks with Ham	*139*
Casseroled Leeks	*140*
Casseroled Celery	*140*
Meat-stuffed Peppers	*141*
Meat-stuffed Peppers with Tomato	*142*
Turkey-stuffed Peppers with Lemon and Thyme	*142*
Polish-style Creamed Mushrooms	*143*
Paprika Mushrooms	*144*
Curried Mushrooms	*144*

Lentil Dhal	145
Dhal with Onions and Tomatoes	147
Vegetable Madras	149
Mixed Vegetable Curry	151
Jellied Mediterranean Salad	153
Jellied Greek Salad	154
Jellied Russian Salad	154
Kohlrabi Salad with Mustardy Mayonnaise	155
Beetroot, Celery and Apple Cups	156
Mock Waldorf Cups	157
Celeriac Salad with Garlic, Mayonnaise and Pistachios	157
Continental Celeriac Salad	158
Celeriac Salad with Bacon	159
Artichoke Salad with Peppers and Eggs in Warm Dressing	160
Sage and Onion Stuffing	161
Celery and Pesto Stuffing	162
Leek and Tomato Stuffing	162
Bacon Stuffing	163
Bacon and Apricot Stuffing	164
Mushroom, Lemon and Thyme Stuffing	164
Mushroom and Leek Stuffing	165
Ham and Pineapple Stuffing	166
Asian Mushroom and Cashew Nut Stuffing	167
Ham and Carrot Stuffing	168
Ham, Banana and Sweetcorn Stuffing	168
Italian Stuffing	169
Spanish Stuffing	170

Orange and Coriander Stuffing	170
Lime and Coriander Stuffing	171
Orange and Apricot Stuffing	172
Apple, Raisin and Walnut Stuffing	173
Apple, Prune and Brazil Nut Stuffing	174
Apple, Date and Hazelnut Stuffing	174
Garlic, Rosemary and Lemon Stuffing	175
Garlic, Rosemary and Lemon Stuffing with Parmesan Cheese	176
Seafood Stuffing	176
Parma Ham Stuffing	177
Sausagemeat Stuffing	177
Sausagemeat and Liver Stuffing	178
Sausagemeat and Sweetcorn Stuffing	178
Sausagemeat and Orange Stuffing	178
Chestnut Stuffing with Egg	179
Chestnut and Cranberry Stuffing	180
Creamy Chestnut Stuffing	180
Creamy Chestnut and Sausagement Stuffing	181
Creamy Chestnut Stuffing with Whole Chestnuts	181
Chestnut Stuffing with Parsley and Thyme	182
Chestnut Stuffing with Gammon	183
Chicken Liver Stuffing	184
Chicken Liver Stuffing with Pecans and Orange	185
Triple Nut Stuffing	185
Potato and Turkey Liver Stuffing	186
Rice Stuffing with Herbs	187
Spanish Rice Stuffing with Tomato	188

Fruited Rice Stuffing	189
Far East Rice Stuffing	190
Savoury Rice Stuffing with Nuts	190
Chocolate Crispies	191
Devil's Food Cake	192
Mocha Torte	193
Multi-layer Cake	194
Black Forest Cherry Torte	194
Chocolate Orange Gateau	195
Chocolate Butter Cream Layer Cake	196
Chocolate Mocha Cake	197
Orange-choc Layer Cake	197
Double Chocolate Cake	197
Whipped Cream and Walnut Torte	198
Christmas Gâteau	199
American Brownies	200
Chocolate Nut Brownies	201
Oaten Toffee Triangles	201
Muesli Triangles	202
Chocolate Queenies	202
Flaky Chocolate Queenies	203
Breakfast Bran and Pineapple Cake	204
Fruited Chocolate Biscuit Crunch Cake	205
Fruited Mocha Biscuit Crunch Cake	206
Fruited Rum and Raisin Biscuit Crunch Cake	206
Fruited Whisky and Orange Biscuit Crunch Cake	206
White Chocolate Fruited Crunch Cake	207

Two-layer Apricot and Raspberry Cheesecake	207
Peanut Butter Cheesecake	210
Lemon Curd Cheesecake	211
Chocolate Cheesecake	211
Sharon Fruit Cheesecake	212
Blueberry Cheesecake	213
Baked Lemon Cheesecake	214
Baked Lime Cheesecake	215
Baked Blackcurrant Cheesecake	215
Baked Raspberry Cheesecake	215
Beef and Pickled Onion	216
Pizza Croissant	216
Cottage Cheese and Lemon	217
Spicy Jam and Banana	217
Chocolate and Banana	217
Baked Beans on Toast	218
Cheesy Beans on Toast	218
Spaghetti on Toast	218
Tipsy Trout	219
Tuna Rarebit with Mayonnaise	219

Braised Beef and Vegetables

Serves 4

30 ml/2 tbsp butter or margarine, at kitchen temperature
1 large onion, grated
3 carrots, thinly sliced
75 g/3 oz mushrooms, thinly sliced
450 g/1 lb rump (tip) steak, cut into small cubes
1 beef stock cube
15 ml/1 tbsp plain (all-purpose) flour
300 ml/½ pt/1¼ cups hot water or beef stock
Freshly ground black pepper
5 ml/1 tsp salt

Put the butter or margarine into a 20 cm/8 in diameter casserole dish (Dutch oven). Melt on Defrost for 45 seconds. Add the vegetables and steak and mix well. Cook, uncovered, on Full for 3 minutes. Crumble in the stock cube and stir in the flour and hot water or stock. Move the mixture to the edge of the dish to form a ring, leaving a small hollow in the centre. Sprinkle with pepper. Cover with clingfilm (plastic wrap) and slit it twice to allow steam to escape. Cook on Full for 9 minutes, turning the dish once. Allow to stand for 5 minutes, then season with the salt and serve.

Beef Stew

Serves 4

450 g/1 lb lean stewing steak, cut into small cubes
15 ml/1 tbsp plain (all-purpose) flour
250 g/9 oz unthawed frozen vegetable stewpack
300 ml/½ pt/1¼ cups boiling water
1 beef stock cube
Freshly ground pepper
2.5–5 ml/½–1 tsp salt

Put the steak in a 23 cm/9 in diameter casserole dish (Dutch oven), not too deep. Sprinkle with the flour, then toss well to coat. Spread out loosely into a single layer. Break up the vegetables, then arrange round the meat. Cover with clingfilm (plastic wrap) and slit it twice to allow steam to escape. Cook on Full for 15 minutes, turning the dish four times. Pour the water over the meat and crumble in the stock cube. Season to taste with pepper and stir thoroughly. Cover as before, then cook on Full for 10 minutes, turning the dish three times. Allow to stand for 5 minutes, then stir round, season with the salt and serve.

Beef and Vegetable Hot-pot

Serves 4

450 g/1 lb potatoes
2 carrots
1 large onion
450 g/1 lb lean stewing steak, cut into small cubes
1 beef stock cube
150 ml/¼ pt/2/3 cup hot beef or vegetable stock
30 ml/2 tbsp butter or margarine

Cut the potatoes, carrots and the onion into transparent wafer-thin slices. Separate the onion slices into rings. Thoroughly grease a 1.75 litre/3 pt/7½ cup dish. Fill with alternate layers of the vegetables and meat, beginning and ending with the potatoes. Cover with clingfilm (plastic wrap) and slit it twice to allow steam to escape. Cook on Full for 15 minutes, turning the dish three times. Crumble the stock cube into the hot stock and stir until dissolved. Pour gently down the side of the dish so it flows through the meat and vegetables. Top with flakes of the butter or margarine. Cover as before and cook on Full for 15 minutes, turning the dish three times. Allow to stand for 5 minutes. Brown under a hot grill (broiler), if liked.

Beef Curry

Serves 4–5

An Anglicised version of a medium-hot curry. Serve with basmati rice and sambals (side dishes) of plain yoghurt, sliced cucumber sprinkled with chopped fresh coriander (cilantro), and chutney.

450 g/1 lb lean stewing beef, cut into small cubes
2 onions, chopped
2 garlic cloves, crushed
15 ml/1 tbsp sunflower or corn oil
30 ml/2 tbsp hot curry powder
30 ml/2 tbsp tomato purée (paste)
15 ml/1 tbsp plain (all-purpose) flour
4 green cardamom pods
15 ml/1 tbsp garam masala
450 ml/¾ pt/2 cups hot water
5 ml/1 tsp salt

Arrange the meat in a single layer in a deep 25 cm/10 in diameter dish. Cover with a plate and cook on Full for 15 minutes, stirring twice. Meanwhile, fry (sauté) the onions and garlic conventionally in the oil in a frying pan (skillet) over a medium heat until pale golden. Stir in the curry powder, tomato purée, flour, cardamom pods and garam masala, then gradually blend in the hot water. Cook, stirring, until the mixture comes to the boil and thickens. Remove the dish of meat from the microwave and stir in the contents of the frying pan. Cover with clingfilm (plastic wrap) and slit it twice to allow steam to escape. Cook on Full for 10 minutes, turning the dish twice. Allow to stand for 5 minutes before serving.

Basic Mince

Serves 4

450 g/1 lb/4 cups lean minced (ground) beef
1 onion, grated
30 ml/2 tbsp plain (all-purpose) flour
450 ml/¾ pt/2 cups hot water
1 beef stock cube
5 ml/1 tsp salt

Place the meat in a deep 20 cm/8 in diameter dish. Thoroughly mix in the onion and flour with a fork. Cook, uncovered, on Full for 5 minutes. Break up the meat with a fork. Add the water and crumble in the stock cube. Stir well to mix. Cover with clingfilm (plastic wrap) and slit it twice to allow steam to escape. Cook on Full for 15 minutes, turning the dish four times. Allow to stand for 4 minutes. Add the salt and stir round before serving.

Cottage Pie

Serves 4

1 quantity Basic Mince
675 g/1½ lb freshly cooked potatoes
30 ml/2 tbsp butter or margarine
60–90 ml/4–6 tbsp hot milk

Cool the Basic Mince to lukewarm and transfer to a greased 1 litre/1¾ pt/4¼ cup pie dish. Cream the potatoes with the butter or margarine and enough of the milk to make a light and fluffy mash. Pipe over the meat mixture or spread smoothly then rough up with a fork. Reheat, uncovered, on Full for 3 minutes. Alternatively, brown under a hot grill (broiler).

Cottage Pie with Cheese

Serves 4

Prepare as for Cottage Pie, but add 50–75 g/2–3 oz/½–¾ cup grated Cheddar cheese to the potatoes after creaming with the butter and hot milk.

Mince with Oats

Serves 4

Prepare as for Basic Mince, but add 1 carrot, grated, with the onion. Substitute 25 g/1 oz/½ cup porridge oats for the flour. Cook for the first time for 7 minutes.

Chilli con Carne

Serves 4–5

450 g/1 lb/4 cups lean minced (ground) beef
1 onion, grated
2 garlic cloves, crushed
5–20 ml/1–4 tsp chilli seasoning
400 g/14 oz/1 large can chopped tomatoes
5 ml/1 tsp Worcestershire sauce
400 g/14 oz/1 large can red kidney beans, drained
5 ml/1 tsp salt
Jacket Potatoes or boiled rice, to serve

Put the beef into a 23 cm/9 in diameter casserole dish (Dutch oven). Stir in the onion and garlic with a fork. Cook, uncovered, on Full for 5 minutes. Break up the meat with a fork. Work in all the remaining ingredients except the salt. Cover with clingfilm (plastic wrap) and slit it twice to allow steam to escape. Cook on Full for 15 minutes, turning the dish three times. Allow to stand for 4 minutes. Season with the salt before serving with jacket potatoes or boiled rice.

Curried Mince

Serves 4

2 onions, grated
2 garlic cloves, crushed
450 g/1 lb/4 cups lean minced (ground) beef
15 ml/1 tbsp plain (all-purpose) flour
5–10 ml/1–2 tbsp mild curry powder
30 ml/2 tbsp fruity chutney
60 ml/4 tbsp tomato purée (paste)
300 ml/½ pt/1¼ cups boiling water
1 beef stock cube
Salt and freshly ground black pepper

Mash together the onions, garlic and beef. Spread into a 20 cm/8 in diameter casserole dish (Dutch oven). Form into a ring round the edge of the dish, leaving small hollow in the centre. Cover with plate and cook on Full for 5 minutes. Break up with fork. Work in the flour, curry powder, chutney and tomato purée. Gradually stir in the water, then crumble in the stock cube. Cover with clingfilm (plastic wrap) and slit it twice to allow steam to escape. Cook on Full for 15 minutes, turning the dish three times. Allow to stand for 4 minutes. Season to taste, then stir round and serve.

Beef Goulash

Serves 6

40 g/1½ oz/3 tbsp butter, margarine or lard
675 g/1½ lb stewing steak, cut into small cubes
2 large onions, grated
1 medium green (bell) pepper, seeded and finely diced
2 garlic cloves, crushed
4 tomatoes, blanched, skinned and chopped
45 ml/3 tbsp tomato purée (paste)
15 ml/1 tbsp paprika
5 ml/1 tsp caraway seeds
5 ml/1 tsp salt
300 ml/½ pt/1¼ cups boiling water
150 ml/¼ pt/2/3 cup soured (dairy sour) cream

Put the fat in a 1.75 litre/3 pt/7½ cup dish. Melt, uncovered, on Full for 1 minute. Mix in the meat, onions, peppers and garlic. Cover with clingfilm (plastic wrap) and slit it twice to allow steam to escape. Cook on Full for 15 minutes, turning the dish four times. Uncover and stir in the tomatoes, tomato purée, paprika and caraway seeds. Cover as before and cook on Full for 15 minutes, turning the dish four times. Season with the salt and gently mix in the boiling water. Ladle into deep plates and top each generously with the cream.

Beef Goulash with Boiled Potatoes

Serves 6

Prepare as for Beef Goulash, but omit the cream and add 2–3 whole boiled potatoes to each serving.

Butter Bean and Beef Stew with Tomatoes

Serves 6

425 g/15 oz/1 large can butter beans
275 g/10 oz/1 can tomato soup
30 ml/2 tbsp dried onions
6 slices braising steak, about 125 g/4 oz each, beaten flat
Salt and freshly ground black pepper

Combine the beans, soup and onions in a 20 cm/8 in diameter casserole dish (Dutch oven). Cover with a plate and cook on Full for 6 minutes, stirring three times. Arrange the steaks round the edge of the dish. Cover with clingfilm (plastic wrap) and slit it twice to allow steam to escape. Cook on Full for 17 minutes, turning the dish three times. Allow to stand for 5 minutes. Uncover and season to taste before serving.

Beef and Tomato Cake

Serves 2–3

275 g/10 oz/2½ cups minced (ground) beef
30 ml/2 tbsp plain (all-purpose) flour
1 egg
5 ml/1 tsp onion powder
150 ml/¼ pt/2/3 cup tomato juice
5 ml/1 tsp soy sauce
5 ml/1 tsp dried oregano
Boiled pasta, to serve

Thoroughly grease a 900 ml/1½ pt/3¾ cup oval pie dish. Mix the beef with all remaining ingredients and spread smoothly into the dish. Cover with clingfilm (plastic wrap) and slit it twice to allow steam to escape. Cook on Full for 7 minutes, turning the dish twice. Allow to stand for 5 minutes. Cut into two or three portions and serve hot with pasta.

Beef and Mushroom Kebabs

Serves 4

24 fresh or dried bay leaves
½ red (bell) pepper, cut into small squares
½ green (bell) pepper, cut into small squares
750 g/1½ lb grilling (broiling) steak, trimmed and cut into 2.5 cm/1 in cubes
175 g/6 oz button mushrooms
50 g/2 oz/¼ cup butter or margarine, at kitchen temperature
5 ml/1 tsp paprika
5 ml/1 tsp Worcestershire sauce
1 garlic clove, crushed
175 g/6 oz/1½ cups rice, boiled

If using dried bay leaves, place in a small dish, add 90 ml/6 tbsp water and cover with a saucer. Heat on Full for 2 minutes to soften. Put the pepper squares into a dish and just cover with water. Cover with a plate and heat on Full for 1 minute to soften. Drain the peppers and bay leaves. Thread the beef, mushrooms, pepper squares and bay leaves on to twelve 10 cm/4 in wooden skewers. Arrange the kebabs like the spokes of a wheel in a deep 25 cm/10 in diameter dish. Put the butter or margarine, paprika, Worcestershire sauce and garlic in a small dish and heat, uncovered, on Full for 1 minute. Brush over the kebabs. Cook, uncovered, on Full for 8 minutes, turning the dish four times. Carefully turn the kebabs over and brush with the rest of the butter mixture. Cook on Full for a further 4 minutes, turning the dish twice. Arrange on a bed of rice and coat with the juices from the dish. Allow three kebabs per person.

Stuffed Lamb

Serves 4

A slightly Middle Eastern approach here. Serve the lamb with warm pitta bread and a green salad dotted with olives and capers.

4 pieces neck of lamb fillet, about 15 cm/6 in long and 675 g/½ lb each

3 large slices white bread with crusts, cubed

1 onion, cut into 6 wedges

45 ml/3 tbsp toasted pine nuts

30 ml/2 tbsp currants

2.5 ml/½ tsp salt

150 g/5 oz/2/3 cup thick Greek plain yoghurt

Ground cinnamon

8 button mushrooms

15 ml/1 tbsp olive oil

Trim the fat from the lamb. Make a lengthways slit in each piece, taking care not to cut right through the meat. Grind up the bread cubes and onion pieces together in a food processor or blender. Scrape out into a bowl and mix in the pine nuts, currants and salt. Spread equal amounts into the lamb pieces and secure with wooden cocktail sticks (toothpicks). Arrange in a square in a deep 25 cm/10 in diameter dish. Smear with all the yoghurt and dust lightly with cinnamon. Stud randomly with the mushrooms and coat thinly with the oil. Cover with clingfilm (plastic wrap) and slit it twice to allow steam to escape.

Cook on Full for 16 minutes, turning the dish four times. Allow to stand for 5 minutes, then serve.

Minted Lamb Kebabs

Serves 6

900 g/2 lb neck of lamb fillet, trimmed
12 large mint leaves
60 ml/4 tbsp thick plain yoghurt
60 ml/4 tbsp tomato ketchup (catsup)
1 garlic clove, crushed
5 ml/1 tsp Worcestershire sauce
6 pitta breads, warmed
Lettuce leaves, tomato and cucumber slices

Cut the meat into 2.5 cm/1 in cubes. Thread on to six wooden skewers alternately with the mint leaves. Arrange like the spokes of a wheel in a deep 25 cm/10 in diameter dish. Thoroughly combine the yoghurt, ketchup, garlic and Worcestershire sauce and brush half the mixture over the kebabs. Cook, uncovered, on Full for 8 minutes, turning the dish twice. Turn the kebabs over and brush with the remaining baste. Cook on Full for a further 8 minutes, turning the dish twice. Allow to stand for 5 minutes. Warm the pitta breads briefly under the grill (broiler) until they puff up, then slice along the long edge to make a pocket. Remove the meat from the skewers and discard the bay leaves. Pack the lamb into the pittas, then add a good helping of the salad to each.

Classic Lamb Kebabs

Serves 6

900 g/2 lb neck of lamb fillet, trimmed
12 large mint leaves
30 ml/2 tbsp butter or margarine
5 ml/1 tsp garlic salt
5 ml/1 tsp Worcestershire sauce
5 ml/1 tsp soy sauce
2.5 ml/½ tsp paprika
6 pitta breads, warmed
Lettuce leaves, tomato and cucumber slices

Cut the meat into 2.5 cm/1 in cubes. Thread on to six wooden skewers alternately with the mint leaves. Arrange like the spokes of a wheel in a deep 25 cm/10 in diameter dish. Melt the butter or margarine on Full for 1 minute, then add the garlic salt, Worcestershire sauce, soy sauce and paprika and mix together thoroughly. Brush half the mixture over the kebabs. Cook, uncovered, on Full for 8 minutes, turning the dish twice. Turn the kebabs over and brush with the remaining baste. Cook on Full for a further 8 minutes, turning the dish twice. Allow to stand for 5 minutes. Warm the pitta breads briefly under the grill (broiler) until they puff up, then slice along the long edge to make a pocket. Remove the meat from the skewers and discard the bay leaves. Pack the lamb into the pittas, then add a good helping of the salad to each.

Middle Eastern Lamb with Fruit

Serves 4–6

This delicately spiced and fruited lamb dish is understated elegance, enhanced by its coating of toasted pine nuts and flaked almonds. Serve with yoghurt and buttery rice.

675 g/1½ lb boned lamb, as lean as possible
5 ml/1 tsp ground cinnamon
2.5 ml/½ tsp ground cloves
30 ml/2 tbsp light soft brown sugar
1 onion, chopped
30 ml/2 tbsp lemon juice
10 ml/2 tsp cornflour (cornstarch)
15 ml/1 tbsp cold water
7.5–10 ml/1½–2 tsp salt
400 g/14 oz/1 large can peach slices in natural or apple juice, drained
30 ml/2 tbsp toasted pine nuts
30 ml/2 tbsp flaked (slivered) almonds

Cut the lamb into small cubes. Place in a 1.75 litre/3 pt/7½ cup casserole dish (Dutch oven). Mix together the spices, sugar, onion and lemon juice and add to the dish. Cover with a plate and cook on Full for 5 minutes, then allow to stand for 5 minutes. Repeat three times, stirring well each time. Mix together the cornflour and water to make a smooth paste. Drain the liquid from the lamb and add the cornflour mixture and salt. Pour over the lamb and stir well to mix. Cook, uncovered, on Full for 2 minutes. Stir in the peach slices and cook, uncovered, on Full for a further 1½ minutes. Sprinkle with the pine nuts and almonds and and serve.

Mock Irish Stew

Serves 4

675 g/1½ lb cubed stewing lamb
2 large onions, coarsely grated
450 g/1 lb potatoes, finely diced
300 ml/½ pt/1¼ cups boiling water
5 ml/1 tsp salt
45 ml/3 tbsp chopped parsley

Trim away any excess fat from the lamb. Place the meat and vegetables in a single layer in a deep 25 cm/10 in diameter dish. Cover with clingfilm (plastic wrap) and slit it twice to allow steam to escape. Cook on Full for 15 minutes, turning the dish twice. Mix the water and salt and pour over the meat and vegetables, stirring thoroughly to combine. Cover as before and cook on Full for 20 minutes, turning the dish three times. Allow to stand for 10 minutes. Uncover and sprinkle with the parsley before serving.

Farmer's Wife Lamb Chops

Serves 4

3 cold cooked potatoes, thinly sliced
3 cold cooked carrots, thinly sliced
4 lean lamb chops, 150 g/5 oz each
1 small onion, grated
1 cooking (tart) apple, peeled and grated
30 ml/2 tbsp apple juice
Salt and freshly ground black pepper
15 ml/1 tbsp butter or margarine

Arrange the potato and carrot slices in a single layer over the base of a deep 20 cm/8 in diameter dish. Arrange the chops on top. Sprinkle with the onion and apple and pour the juice over. Season to taste and dot with flakes of the butter or margarine. Cover with clingfilm (plastic wrap) and slit it twice to allow steam to escape. Cook on Full for 15 minutes, turning the dish twice. Allow to stand for 5 minutes before serving.

Lamb Hot-pot

Serves 4

675 g/1½ lb potatoes, very thinly sliced
2 onions, very thinly sliced
3 carrots, very thinly sliced
2 large celery stalks, cut diagonally into thin strips
8 best end of neck lamb chops, about 1 kg/2 lb in all
1 beef stock cube
300 ml/½ pt/1¼ cups boiling water
5 ml/1 tsp salt
25 ml/1½ tbsp melted butter or margarine

Arrange half the prepared vegetables in layers in a lightly greased 2.25 litre/4 pt/10 cup casserole dish (Dutch oven). Place the chops on top and cover with the remaining vegetables. Cover with clingfilm (plastic wrap) and slit it twice to allow steam to escape. Cook on Full for 15 minutes, turning the dish three times. Remove from the microwave and uncover. Crumble the stock cube into the water and add the salt. Pour gently down the side of the casserole. Trickle the butter or margarine over the top. Cover as before and cook on Full for 15 minutes. Allow to stand for 6 minutes before serving.

Lamb Loaf with Mint and Rosemary

Serves 4

450 g/1 lb/4 cups minced (ground) lamb
1 garlic clove, crushed
2.5 ml/½ tsp dried crumbled rosemary
2.5 ml/½ tsp dried mint
30 ml/2 tbsp plain (all-purpose) flour
2 large eggs, beaten
2.5 ml/½ tsp salt
5 ml/1 tsp brown table sauce
Grated nutmeg

Lightly grease a 900 ml/1½ pt/3¾ cup oval pie dish. Mix together all the ingredients except the nutmeg and spread smoothly into the dish. Cover with clingfilm (plastic wrap) and slit it twice to allow steam to escape. Cook on Full for 8 minutes, turning the dish twice. Allow to stand for 4 minutes, then uncover and sprinkle with nutmeg. Cut into portions to serve.

Lamb Bredie with Tomatoes

Serves 6

Prepare as for Chicken Bredie with Tomatoes, but substitute boned and coarsely chopped lamb for the chicken.

Lamb Biriani

Serves 4–6

5 cardamom pods
30 ml/2 tbsp sunflower oil
450 g/1 lb trimmed neck of lamb fillet, cut into small cubes
2 garlic cloves, crushed
20 ml/4 tsp garam masala
225 g/8 oz/1¼ cups easy-cook long-grain rice
600 ml/1 pt/2½ cups hot chicken stock
10 ml/2 tsp salt
125 g/4 oz/1 cup flaked (slivered) almonds, toasted

Split the cardamom pods to remove the seeds, then crush the seeds with a pestle and mortar. Heat the oil in a 1.5 litre/3 pt/7½ cup casserole dish (Dutch oven) on Full for 1½ minutes. Add the lamb, garlic, cardamom seeds and garam masala. Mix well, then arrange round the edge of the dish, leaving a small hollow in the centre. Cover with clingfilm (plastic wrap) and slit it twice to allow steam to escape. Cook on Full for 10 minutes. Uncover and mix in the rice, stock and salt. Cover as before and cook on Full for 15 minutes. Allow to stand for 3 minutes, then spoon out on to warmed plates and sprinkle each portion with the almonds.

Ornate Biriani

Serves 4–6

Prepare as for Lamb Biriani, but arrange the biriani on a warmed serving dish and garnish with chopped hard-boiled (hard-cooked) eggs, tomato wedges, coriander (cilantro) leaves and fried (sautéed) chopped onion.

Moussaka

Serves 6–8

You require a little patience to prepare this multi-layered lamb-based Greek classic but the results are well worth the effort. Poached aubergine (eggplant) slices makes this less rich and easier to digest than some versions.

For the aubergine layers:
675 g/1½ lb aubergines
75 ml/5 tbsp hot water
5 ml/1 tsp salt
15 ml/1 tbsp fresh lemon juice

For the meat layers:
40 g/1½ oz/3 tbsp butter, margarine or olive oil
2 onions, finely chopped
1 garlic clove, crushed
350 g/12 oz/3 cups cold cooked minced (ground) lamb
125 g/4 oz/2 cups fresh white breadcrumbs
Salt and freshly ground black pepper
4 tomatoes, blanched, skinned and sliced

For the sauce:
425 ml/¾ pt/scant 2 cups full-cream milk
40 g/1½ oz/3 tbsp butter or margarine
45 ml/3 tbsp plain (all-purpose) flour

75 g/3 oz/¾ cup Cheddar cheese, grated

1 egg yolk

Moussaka with Potatoes

Serves 6–8

Prepare as for Moussaka, but substitute sliced cooked potatoes for the aubergines (eggplants).

Quick Moussaka

Serves 3–4

A quick alternative with an acceptable flavour and texture.

1 aubergine (eggplant), about 225 g/8 oz
15 ml/1 tbsp cold water
300 ml/½ pt/1¼ cups cold milk
300 ml/½ pt/1¼ cups water
1 packet instant mashed potato to serve 4
225 g/8 oz/2 cups cold cooked minced (ground) lamb
5 ml/1 tsp dried marjoram
5 ml/1 tsp salt
2 garlic cloves, crushed
3 tomatoes, blanched, skinned and sliced
150 ml/¼ pt/2/3 cup thick Greek plain yoghurt
1 egg
Salt and freshly ground black pepper
50 g/2 oz/½ cup Cheddar cheese, grated

Top and tail the aubergine and halve it lengthways. Place in a shallow dish, cut sides uppermost and sprinkle with the cold water. Cover with clingfilm (plastic wrap) and slit it twice to allow steam to escape. Cook on Full for 5½–6 minutes until tender. Allow to stand for 2 minutes, then drain. Pour the milk and water into a bowl and stir in the dried potato. Cover with a plate and cook on Full for 6 minutes. Stir well, then mix in the lamb, marjoram, salt and garlic. Slice the unpeeled aubergine. Arrange alternate layers of aubergine slices and the potato mixture in a 2.25 litre/4 pt/10 cup greased casserole dish (Dutch oven), using half the tomato slices to form a 'sandwich filling' in the centre. Cover with the remaining tomato slices. Beat together the yoghurt and egg and season to taste. Spoon over the tomatoes and sprinkle with the cheese. Cover with clingfilm as before. Cook on Full for 7 minutes. Uncover and brown under a hot grill (broiler) before serving.

Lamb Mince

Serves 4

Prepare as for Basic Mince, but substitute minced (ground) lamb for the minced beef.

Shepherd's Pie

Serves 4

Prepare as for Basic Mince, but substitute lamb mince for beef. Cool to lukewarm, then transfer to a 1 litre/1¾ pt/4½ cup greased pie dish. Top with 750 g/1½ lb hot mashed potato creamed with 15–30 ml/1–2 tbsp butter or margarine and 60 ml/4 tbsp hot milk. Season well with salt and freshly ground black pepper. Spread over the meat mixture, then rough up with a fork. Reheat, uncovered, on Full for 2–3 minutes or brown under a hot grill (broiler).

Country Liver in Red Wine

Serves 4

25 g/1 oz/2 tbsp butter or margarine
2 onions, grated
450 g/1 lb lambs' liver, cut into narrow strips
15 ml/1 tbsp plain (all-purpose) flour
300 ml/½ pt/1¼ cups red wine
15 ml/1 tbsp dark soft brown sugar
1 beef stock cube, crumbled
30 ml/2 tbsp chopped parsley
Salt and freshly ground black pepper
Buttered boiled potatoes and lightly cooked shredded cabbage, to serve

Put the butter or margarine in a deep 25 cm/10 in diameter dish. Melt, uncovered, on Defrost for 2 minutes. Stir in the onions and liver. Cover with a plate and cook on Full for 5 minutes. Mix in all the remaining ingredients except the salt and pepper. Cover with a plate and cook on Full for 6 minutes, stirring twice. Allow to stand for 3 minutes. Season to taste and serve with buttered boiled potatoes and cabbage.

Liver and Bacon

Serves 4–6

2 onions, grated
8 bacon rashers (slices), coarsely chopped
450 g/1 lb lambs' liver, cut into small cubes
45 ml/3 tbsp cornflour (cornstarch)
60 ml/4 tbsp cold water
150 ml/¼ pt/2/3 cup boiling water
Salt and freshly ground black pepper

Put the onions and bacon in a 1.75 litre/3 pt/7½ cup casserole dish (Dutch oven). Cook, uncovered, on Full for 7 minutes, stirring twice. Mix in the liver. Cover with a plate and cook on Full for 8 minutes, stirring three times. Mix the cornflour with the cold water to make a smooth paste. Stir into the liver and onions, then gradually blend in the boiling water. Cover with a plate and cook on Full for 6 minutes, stirring three times. Allow to stand for 4 minutes. Season to taste and serve.

Liver and Bacon with Apple

Serves 4–6

Prepare as for Liver and Bacon, but substitute 1 eating (dessert) apple, peeled and grated, for one of the onions. Substitute apple juice at room temperature for half the boiling water.

Kidneys in Red Wine with Brandy

Serves 4

6 lambs' kidneys
30 ml/2 tbsp butter or margarine
1 onion, finely chopped
30 ml/2 tbsp plain (all-purpose) flour
150 ml/¼ pt/2/3 cup dry red wine
2 beef stock cubes
50 g/2 oz mushrooms, sliced
10 ml/2 tsp tomato purée (paste)
2.5 ml/½ tsp paprika
2.5 ml/½ tsp mustard powder
30 ml/2 tbsp chopped parsley
30 ml/2 tbsp brandy

Skin and halve the kidneys, then cut out and discard the cores with a sharp knife. Slice very thinly. Melt half the butter, uncovered, on Defrost for 1 minute. Stir in the kidneys and set aside. Put the remaining butter and the onion in a 1.5 litre/2½ pt/6 cup dish. Cook, uncovered, on Full for 2 minutes, stirring once. Mix in the flour, then the wine. Cook, uncovered, on Full for 3 minutes, stirring briskly every minute. Crumble in the stock cubes, then stir in the mushrooms, tomato purée, paprika, mustard and the kidneys with the butter or margarine. Mix thoroughly. Cover with clingfilm (plastic wrap) and slit it twice to allow steam to escape. Cook on Full for 5 minutes, turning the dish once. Allow to stand for 3 minutes, then uncover and sprinkle with the parsley. Warm the brandy in a cup on Full for 10–15 seconds. Pour over the kidney mixture and ignite. Serve when the flames have subsided.

Venison Steaks with Oyster Mushrooms and Blue Cheese

Serves 4

Salt and freshly ground black pepper
8 small venison steaks
5 ml/1 tsp juniper berries, crushed
5 ml/1 tsp herbes de Provence
30 ml/2 tbsp olive oil
300 ml/½ pt/1¼ cups dry red wine
60 ml/4 tbsp rich beef stock
60 ml/4 tbsp gin
1 onion, chopped
225 g/8 oz oyster mushrooms, trimmed and sliced
250 ml/8 fl oz/1 cup single (light) cream
30 ml/2 tbsp redcurrant jelly (clear conserve)
60 ml/4 tbsp blue cheese, crumbled
30 ml/2 tbsp chopped parsley

Season the venison to taste, then work in the juniper berries and herbes de Provence. Heat the oil in a browning dish on Full for 2 minutes. Add the steaks and cook, uncovered, on Full for 3 minutes, turning once. Add the wine, stock, gin, onion, mushrooms, cream and redcurrant jelly. Cover with clingfilm (plastic wrap) and slit it twice to allow steam to escape. Cook on Medium for 25 minutes, turning the dish four times. Mix in the cheese. Cover with a heatproof plate and cook on Full for 2 minutes. Allow to stand for 3 minutes, then uncover and serve garnished with the parsley.

Cooking Small Pasta

Follow the directions for cooking large pasta but cook for only 4–5 minutes. Cover and stand for 3 minutes, then drain and serve.

Chinese Noodle and Mushroom Salad with Walnuts

Serves 6

30 ml/2 tbsp sesame oil
175 g/6 oz mushrooms, sliced
250 g/9 oz thread egg noodles
7.5 ml/1½ tsp salt
75 g/3 oz/¾ cup chopped walnuts
5 spring onions (scallions), chopped
30 ml/2 tbsp soy sauce

Heat the oil, uncovered, on Defrost for 2½ minutes. Add the mushrooms. Cover with a plate and cook on Full for 3 minutes, stirring twice. Set aside. Put the noodles in a large bowl and add enough boiling water to come 5 cm/2 in above the level of the pasta. Stir in the salt. Cook, uncovered, on Full for 4–5 minutes until the noodles swell and are just tender. Drain and allow to cool. Mix in the remaining ingredients including the mushrooms and toss well to mix.

Pepper Macaroni

Serves 2

300 ml/½ pt/1¼ cups tomato juice
125 g/4 oz/1 cup elbow macaroni
5 ml/1 tsp salt
30 ml/2 tbsp white wine, heated
1 small red or green (bell) pepper, seeded and chopped
45 ml/3 tbsp olive oil
75 g/3 oz/¾ cup Gruyère (Swiss) or Emmental cheese, grated
30 ml/2 tbsp chopped parsley

Pour the tomato juice into a 1.25 litre/2¼ pt/5½ cup dish. Cover with a plate and heat on Full for 3½–4 minutes until very hot and bubbling. Stir in all the remaining ingredients except the cheese and parsley. Cover as before and cook on Full for 10 minutes, stirring twice. Allow to stand for 5 minutes. Sprinkle with the cheese and parsley. Reheat, uncovered, on Full for about 1 minute until the cheese melts.

Family Macaroni Cheese

Serves 6–7

For convenience, this recipe is for a large family-sized meal, but any leftovers can be reheated in portions in the microwave.

350 g/12 oz/3 cups elbow macaroni
10 ml/2 tsp salt
30 ml/2 tbsp cornflour (cornstarch)
600 ml/1 pt/2½ cups cold milk
1 egg, beaten
10 ml/2 tsp made mustard
Freshly ground black pepper
275 g/10 oz/2½ cups Cheddar cheese, grated

Put the macaroni in a deep dish. Stir in the salt and sufficient boiling water to come 5 cm/2 in above the level of the pasta. Cook, uncovered, on Full for about 10 minutes until just tender, stirring three times. Drain if necessary, then leave to stand while preparing the sauce. In a separate large bowl, mix the cornflour smoothly with some of the cold milk, then mix in the remainder. Cook, uncovered, on Full for 6–7 minutes until smoothly thickened, whisking every minute. Mix in the egg, mustard and pepper followed by two-thirds of the cheese and all the macaroni. Mix thoroughly with a fork. Spread evenly into a buttered 30 cm/12 in diameter dish. Sprinkle the remaining cheese over the top. Reheat, uncovered, on Full for 4–5 minutes. If liked, brown quickly under a hot grill (broiler) before serving.

Classic Macaroni Cheese

Serves 4–5

This version is slightly richer than Family Macaroni Cheese and lends itself to a number of variations.

225 g/8 oz/2 cups elbow macaroni
7.5 ml/1½ tsp salt
30 ml/2 tbsp butter or margarine
30 ml/2 tbsp plain (all-purpose) flour
300 ml/½ pt/1¼ cups milk
225 g/8 oz/2 cups Cheddar cheese, grated
5–10 ml/1–2 tsp made mustard
Salt and freshly ground black pepper

Put the macaroni in a deep dish. Stir in the salt and sufficient boiling water to come 5 cm/2 in above the level of the pasta. Cook, uncovered, on Full for 8–10 minutes until just tender, stirring two or three times. Stand for 3–4 minutes inside the microwave. Drain if necessary, then leave to stand while preparing the sauce. Melt the butter or margarine, uncovered, on Defrost for 1–1½ minutes. Stir in the flour, then gradually blend in the milk. Cook, uncovered, on Full for 6–7 minutes until smoothly thickened, whisking every minute. Mix in two-thirds of the cheese, followed by the mustard and seasoning, then the macaroni. Spread evenly in a 20 cm/8 in diameter dish. Sprinkle with the remaining cheese. Reheat, uncovered, on Full for 3–4 minutes. If liked, brown quickly under a hot grill (broiler) before serving.

Macaroni Cheese with Stilton

Serves 4–5

Prepare as for Classic Macaroni Cheese, but substitute 100 g/3½ oz/1 cup crumbled Stilton for half the Cheddar cheese.

Macaroni Cheese with Bacon

Serves 4–5

Prepare as for Classic Macaroni Cheese, but stir in 6 rashers (slices) streaky bacon, grilled (broiled) until crisp then crumbled, with the mustard and seasoning.

Macaroni Cheese with Tomatoes

Serves 4–5

Prepare as for Classic Macaroni Cheese, but place a layer of tomato slices from about 3 skinned tomatoes on top of the pasta before sprinkling with the remaining cheese.

Spaghetti Carbonara

Serves 4

75 ml/5 tbsp double (heavy) cream
2 large eggs
100 g/4 oz/1 cup Parma ham, chopped
175 g/6 oz/1½ cups grated Parmesan cheese
350 g/12 oz spaghetti or other large pasta

Beat together the cream and eggs. Stir in the ham and 90 ml/6 tbsp of the Parmesan. Cook the spaghetti as directed. Drain and place in a serving dish. Add the cream mixture and toss all together with two wooden forks or spoons. Cover with kitchen paper and reheat on Full for 1½ minutes. Serve each portion topped with the remaining Parmesan.

Pizza-style Macaroni Cheese

Serves 4–5

225 g/8 oz/2 cups elbow macaroni
7.5 ml/1½ tsp salt
30 ml/2 tbsp butter or margarine
30 ml/2 tbsp plain (all-purpose) flour
300 ml/½ pt/1¼ cups milk
125 g/4 oz/1 cup Cheddar cheese, grated
125 g/4 oz/1 cup Mozzarella cheese, grated
5–10 ml/1–2 tsp made mustard
Salt and freshly ground black pepper
212 g/7 oz/1 small can tuna in oil, drained and oil reserved
12 stoned (pitted) black olives, sliced
1 canned pimiento, sliced
2 tomatoes, blanched, skinned and coarsely chopped
5–10 ml/1–2 tsp red or green pesto (optional)
Basil leaves, to garnish

Put the macaroni in a deep dish. Stir in the salt and sufficient boiling water to come 5 cm/2 in above the level of the pasta. Cook, uncovered, on Full for 8–10 minutes until just tender, stirring two or three times. Stand for 3–4 minutes inside the microwave. Drain if necessary, then leave to stand while preparing the sauce. Melt the butter or margarine, uncovered, on Defrost for 1–1½ minutes. Stir in the flour, then gradually blend in the milk. Cook, uncovered, on Full for 6–7 minutes until smoothly thickened, whisking every minute. Mix in two-thirds of each cheese, followed by the mustard and seasoning. Stir in the macaroni, tuna, 15 ml/1 tbsp of the tuna oil, the olives, pimiento, tomatoes and pesto, if using. Spread evenly in a 20 cm/8 in diameter dish. Sprinkle with the remaining cheeses. Reheat, uncovered, on Full for 3–4 minutes. If liked, brown quickly under a hot grill (broiler) before serving garnished with basil leaves.

Spaghetti Cream with Spring Onions

Serves 4

150 ml/¼ pt/2/3 cup double (heavy) cream
1 egg yolk
150 g/5 oz/1¼ cups grated Parmesan cheese
8 spring onions (scallions), finely chopped
Salt and freshly ground black pepper
350 g/12 oz spaghetti or other large pasta

Beat together the cream, egg yolk, 45 ml/3 tbsp of the Parmesan and the spring onions. Season well to taste. Cook the spaghetti as directed. Drain and place in a serving dish. Add the cream mixture and toss all together with two wooden forks or spoons. Cover with kitchen paper and reheat on Full for 1½ minutes. Offer the remaining Parmesan cheese separately.

Spaghetti Bolognese

Serves 4–6

450 g/1 lb/4 cups lean minced (ground) beef
1 garlic clove, crushed
1 large onion, grated
1 green (bell) pepper, seeded and finely chopped
5 ml/1 tsp Italian seasoning or dried mixed herbs
400 g/14 oz/1 large can chopped tomatoes
45 ml/3 tbsp tomato purée (paste)
1 beef stock cube
75 ml/5 tbsp red wine or water
15 ml/1 tbsp dark soft brown sugar
5 ml/1 tsp salt
Freshly ground black pepper
350 g/12 oz freshly cooked and drained spaghetti or other pasta
Grated Parmesan cheese

Combine the beef with the garlic in a 1.75 litre/3 pt/7½ cup dish. Cook, uncovered, on Full for 5 minutes. Mix in all the remaining ingredients except the salt, pepper and spaghetti. Cover with a plate and cook on Full for 15 minutes, stirring four times with a fork to break up the meat. Allow to stand for 4 minutes. Season with the salt and pepper to taste and serve with the spaghetti. Offer the Parmesan cheese separately.

Spaghetti with Turkey Bolognese Sauce

Serves 4

Prepare as for Spaghetti Bolognese, but substitute minced (ground) turkey for the beef.

Spaghetti with Ragu Sauce

Serves 4

A traditional and economical sauce, first used in England in Soho trattorias shortly after World War Two.

20 ml/4 tsp olive oil
1 large onion, finely chopped
1 garlic clove, crushed
1 small carrot, grated
250 g/8 oz/2 cups lean minced (ground) beef
10 ml/2 tsp plain (all-purpose) flour
15 ml/1 tbsp tomato purée (paste)
300 m/½ pt/1¼ cups beef stock
45 ml/3 tbsp dry white wine
1.5 ml/¼ tsp dried basil
1 small bay leaf
175 g/6 oz mushrooms, coarsely chopped
Salt and freshly ground black pepper
350 g/12 oz freshly cooked and drained spaghetti or other pasta
Grated Parmesan cheese

Place the oil, onion, garlic and carrot in a 1.75 litre/3 pt/7½ cup dish. Heat, uncovered, on Full for 6 minutes. Add all the remaining ingredients except the salt, pepper and spaghetti. Cover with a plate and cook on Full for 11 minutes, stirring three times. Allow to stand for 4 minutes. Season with salt and pepper, remove the bay leaf and serve with the spaghetti. Offer the Parmesan cheese separately.

Spaghetti with Butter

Serves 4

350 g/12 oz pasta
60 ml/4 tbsp butter or olive oil
Grated Parmesan cheese

Cook the pasta as directed. Drain and place in a large dish with the butter or olive oil. Toss with two spoons until the pasta is well coated. Spoon on to four warmed plates and heap grated Parmesan cheese on each.

Pasta with Garlic

Serves 4

350 g/12 oz pasta
2 cloves garlic, crushed
50 g/2 oz butter
10 ml/2 tsp olive oil
30 ml/2 tbsp chopped parsley
Grated Parmesan cheese
Rocket or radicchio leaves, shredded

Cook the pasta as directed. Heat the garlic, butter and oil on Full for 1½ minutes. Stir in the parsley. Drain the pasta and place in a serving dish. Add the garlic mixture and toss all together with two wooden spoons. Serve straight away sprinkled with Parmesan and garnished with shredded rocket or radicchio leaves.

Spaghetti with Beef and Mixed Vegetable Bolognese Sauce

Serves 4

30 ml/2 tbsp olive oil

1 large onion, finely chopped

2 garlic cloves, crushed

4 rashers (slices) streaky bacon, chopped

1 celery stalk, chopped

1 carrot, grated

125 g/4 oz button mushrooms, thinly sliced

225 g/8 oz/2 cups lean minced (ground) beef

30 ml/2 tbsp plain (all-purpose) flour

1 wine glass dry red wine

150 ml/¼ pt/2/3 cup passata (sieved tomatoes)

60 ml/4 tbsp beef stock

2 large tomatoes, blanched, skinned and chopped

15 ml/1 tbsp dark soft brown sugar

1.5 ml/¼ tsp grated nutmeg

15 ml/1 tbsp chopped basil leaves

Salt and freshly ground black pepper

350 g/12 oz freshly cooked and drained spaghetti

Grated Parmesan cheese

Put the oil, onion, garlic, bacon, celery and carrot in a 2 litre/3½ pt/8½ cup dish. Add the mushrooms and meat. Cook, uncovered, on Full for 6 minutes, stirring twice with a fork to break up the meat. Mix in all the remaining ingredients except the salt, pepper and spaghetti. Cover with a plate and cook on Full for 13–15 minutes, stirring three times. Allow to stand for 4 minutes. Season with salt and pepper and serve with the pasta. Offer the Parmesan cheese separately.

Spaghetti with Meat Sauce and Cream

Serves 4

Prepare as for Spaghetti with Beef and Mixed Vegetable Bolognese Sauce, but stir in 30–45 ml/2–3 tbsp double (heavy) cream at the end.

Spaghetti with Marsala Meat Sauce

Serves 4

Prepare as for Spaghetti with Beef and Mixed Vegetable Bolognese Sauce, but substitute marsala for the wine and add 45 ml/3 tbsp Marscapone cheese at the end.

Pasta alla Marinara

Serves 4

This means 'sailor style' and comes from Naples.
30 ml/2 tbsp olive oil
3–4 garlic cloves, crushed
8 large tomatoes, blanched, skinned and chopped
5 ml/1 tsp finely chopped mint
15 ml/1 tbsp finely chopped basil leaves
Salt and freshly ground black pepper
350 g/12 oz freshly cooked and drained pasta
Grated Pecorino or Parmesan cheese, to serve

Put all the ingredients except the pasta in a 1.25 litre/2¼ pt/5½ cup dish. Cover with a plate and cook on Full for 6–7 minutes, stirring three times. Serve with the pasta and offer the Pecorino or Parmesan cheese separately.

Pasta Matriciana

Serves 4

A rustic pasta sauce from the central Abruzzo region in Italy.

30 ml/2 tbsp olive oil
1 onion, chopped
5 rashers (slices) unsmoked streaky bacon, coarsely chopped
8 tomatoes, blanched, skinned and chopped
2–3 garlic cloves, crushed
350 g/12 oz freshly cooked and drained pasta
Grated Pecorino or Parmesan cheese, to serve

Put all the ingredients except the pasta in a 1.25 litre/2¼ pt/5½ cup dish. Cover with a plate and cook on Full for 6 minutes, stirring twice. Serve with the pasta and offer the Pecorino or Parmesan cheese separately.

Pasta with Tuna and Capers

Serves 4

15 ml/1 tbsp butter
200 g/7 oz/1 small can tuna in oil
60 ml/4 tbsp vegetable stock or white wine
15 ml/1 tbsp capers, chopped
30 ml/2 tbsp chopped parsley
350 g/12 oz freshly cooked and drained pasta
Grated Parmesan cheese

Put the butter in a 600 ml/1 pt/2½ cup dish and melt, uncovered, on Defrost for 1½ minutes. Add the contents of the can of tuna and flake the fish. Stir in the stock or wine, capers and parsley. Cover with a plate and heat on Full for 3–4 minutes. Serve with the pasta and offer the Parmesan cheese separately.

Pasta Napoletana

Serves 4

This flamboyant tomato sauce from Naples, with a warm and colourful flavour, is best made in summer when tomatoes are at their most abundant.

8 large ripe tomatoes, blanched, skinned and coarsely chopped
30 ml/2 tbsp olive oil
1 onion, chopped
2–4 garlic cloves, crushed
1 celery stalk, finely chopped
15 ml/1 tbsp chopped basil leaves
10 ml/2 tsp light soft brown sugar
60 ml/4 tbsp water or red wine
Salt and freshly ground black pepper
30 ml/2 tbsp chopped parsley
350 g/12 oz freshly cooked and drained pasta
Grated Parmesan cheese

Put the tomatoes, oil, onion, garlic, celery, basil, sugar and water or wine in a 1.25 litre/2¼ pt/5½ cup dish. Mix well. Cover with a plate and cook on Full for 7 minutes, stirring twice. Season to taste, then stir in the parsley. Serve straight away with the pasta and offer the Parmesan cheese separately.

Pasta Pizzaiola

Serves 4

Prepare as for Pasta Napoletana, but increase the tomatoes to 10, omit the onion, celery and water and use double the amount of parsley. Add 15 ml/1 tbsp fresh or 2.5 ml/½ tsp dried oregano with the parsley.

Pasta with Peas

Serves 4

Prepare as for Pasta Napoletana, but add 125 g/4 oz/1 cup coarsely chopped ham and 175 g/6 oz/1½ cups fresh peas to the tomatoes with the other ingredients. Cook for 9–10 minutes.

Pasta with Chicken Liver Sauce

Serves 4

225 g/8 oz chicken livers
30 ml/2 tbsp plain (all-purpose) flour
15 ml/1 tbsp butter
15 ml/1 tbsp olive oil
1–2 garlic cloves, crushed
125 g/4 oz mushrooms, sliced
150 ml/¼ pt/2/3 cup hot water
150 ml/¼ pt/2/3 cup dry red wine
Salt and freshly ground black pepper
350 g/12 oz pasta, freshly cooked and drained

Pasta with Anchovies

Serves 4

30 ml/2 tbsp olive oil
15 ml/1 tbsp butter
2 garlic cloves, crushed
50 g/2 oz/1 small can anchovy fillets in oil
45 ml/3 tbsp chopped parsley
2.5 ml/½ tsp dried basil
Freshly ground black pepper
350 g/12 oz freshly cooked and drained pasta

Put the oil, butter and garlic in a 600 ml/1 pt/2½ cup dish. Chop the anchovies and add with the oil from the can. Mix in the parsley, basil and pepper to taste. Cover with a plate and cook on Full for 3–3½ minutes. Serve straight away with the pasta.

Ravioli with Sauce

Serves 4

350 g/12 oz/3 cups ravioli

Cook as for large pasta, then serve with any of the tomato-based pasta sauces above.

Tortellini

Serves 4

Allow about 250 g/9 oz bought tortellini and cook as for large fresh or dried pasta. Drain thoroughly, add 25 g/1 oz/2 tbsp unsalted (sweet) butter and toss thoroughly. Serve each portion dusted with grated Parmesan cheese.

Lasagne

Serves 4–6

45 ml/3 tbsp hot water
Spaghetti Bolognese sauce
9–10 sheets no-need-to-precook plain, green (verdi) or brown (wholewheat) lasagne
Cheese Sauce
25 g/1 oz/¼ cup grated Parmesan cheese
30 ml/2 tbsp butter
Grated nutmeg

Oil or butter a 20 cm/8 in square dish. Add the hot water to the Bolognese sauce. Place a layer of lasagne sheets in the bottom of the dish, then a layer of Bolognese sauce, then a layer of cheese sauce. Continue with the layers, finishing with the cheese sauce. Sprinkle with the Parmesan cheese, dot with the butter and dust with nutmeg. Cook, uncovered, for 15 minutes, turning the dish twice. Allow to stand for 5 minutes, then continue to cook for a further 15 minutes or until the lasagne feels soft when a knife is pushed through the centre. (The cooking time will vary depending on the initial temperature of the two sauces.)

Pizza Napoletana

Makes 4

The microwave does a great job on pizzas, reminiscent of the ones you can find all over Italy and in Naples in particular.

30 ml/2 tbsp olive oil
2 onions, peeled and finely chopped
1 garlic clove, crushed
150 g/5 oz/2/3 cup tomato purée (paste)
Basic White or Brown Bread Dough
350 g/12 oz/3 cups Mozzarella cheese, grated
10 ml/2 tsp dried oregano
50 g/2 oz/1 small can anchovy fillets in oil

Cook the oil, onions and garlic, uncovered, on Full for 5 minutes, stirring twice. Mix in the tomato purée and set aside. Divide the dough equally into four pieces. Roll each into a round large enough to cover an oiled and floured 20 cm/8 in flat plate. Cover with kitchen paper and leave to stand for 30 minutes. Spread each with the tomato mixture. Mix the cheese with the oregano and sprinkle equally over each pizza. Garnish with the anchovies. Bake individually, covered with kitchen paper, on Full for 5 minutes, turning twice. Eat straight away.

Pizza Margherita

Makes 4

Prepare as for Pizza Napoletana, but substitute dried basil for the oregano and omit the anchovies.

Seafood Pizza

Makes 4

Prepare as for Pizza Napoletana. When cooked, stud with prawns (shrimp), mussels, clams etc.

Pizza Siciliana

Makes 4

Prepare as for Pizza Napoletana. When cooked, stud with 18 small black olives between the anchovies.

Mushroom Pizza

Makes 4

Prepare as for Pizza Napoletana, but sprinkle 100 g/3½ oz thinly sliced mushrooms over the tomato mixture before adding the cheese and herbs. Cook for an extra 30 seconds.

Ham and Pineapple Pizza

Makes 4

Prepare as for Pizza Napoletana, but sprinkle 125 g/4 oz/1 cup chopped ham over the tomato mixture before adding the cheese and herbs. Chop 2 canned pineapple rings and scatter over the top of the pizza. Cook for an extra 45 seconds.

Pepperoni Pizzas

Makes 4

Prepare as for Pizza Napoletana, but top each pizza with 6 thin slices of pepperoni sausage.

Buttered Flaked Almonds

A splendid topping for sweet and savoury dishes.

15 ml/1 tbsp unsalted (sweet) butter
50 g/2 oz/½ cup flaked (slivered) almonds
Plain or flavoured salt or caster (superfine) sugar

Put the butter in a shallow 20 cm/8 in diameter dish. Melt, uncovered, on Full for 45–60 seconds. Add the almonds and cook, uncovered, on Full for 5–6 minutes until golden brown, stirring and turning every minute. Sprinkle with salt for topping savoury dishes, caster sugar for sweet.

Flaked Almonds in Garlic Butter

Prepare as for Buttered Flaked Almonds, but use bought garlic butter. This makes a smart topping for dishes like mashed potato and can also be added to creamy soups.

Dried Chestnuts

The microwave enables dried chestnuts to be cooked and usable in under 2 hours without soaking overnight followed by prolonged cooking. Also the hard job of peeling has already been done for you.

Wash 250 g/8 oz/2 cups dried chestnuts. Put into a 1.75 litre/3 pt/7½ cup dish. Stir in 600 ml/1 pt/2½ cups boiling water. Cover with a plate and cook on Full for 15 minutes, turning the dish three times. Stand in the microwave for 15 minutes. Repeat with the same cooking and standing times. Uncover, add a further 150 ml/¼ pt/2/3 cup boiling water and stir round. Cover as before and cook on Full for 10 minutes, stirring twice. Allow to stand for 15 minutes before using.

Drying Herbs

If you grow your own herbs but find it difficult to dry them in a damp and unpredictable climate, the microwave will do the job for you effectively, efficiently and cleanly in next to no time, so your annual crop can be savoured through the winter months. Each variety of herb should be dried by itself to keep the flavour intact. If you want to later on, you can make up your own blends by mixing several dried herbs together.

Start by cutting the herbs off their shrubs with secateurs or scissors. Pull the leaves (needles in the case of rosemary) off the stalks and pack them loosely into a 300 ml/½ pt/1¼ cup measuring jug, filling it almost to overflowing. Tip into a colander (strainer) and rinse them quickly and gently under cold running water. Drain thoroughly, then dry between the folds of a clean, dry tea towel (dish cloth). Put on top of a double thickness of kitchen paper placed directly on the microwave turntable. Heat, uncovered, on Full for 5–6 minutes, carefully moving the herbs about on the paper two or three times. As soon as they sound like autumn leaves rustling and have lost their bright green colour, you can assume the herbs are dried through. If not, continue to heat for 1–1½ minutes. Remove from the oven and allow to cool. Crush the dried herbs by rubbing them between your hands.

Transfer to airtight jars with stoppers and label. Store away from bright light.

Crisping Breadcrumbs

High-quality pale breadcrumbs – as opposed to marigold-yellow packet ones – are made perfectly in the microwave and turn crisp and brittle without browning. The bread can be fresh or stale but fresh will take a little longer to dry. Crumble 3½ large slices of white or brown bread with crusts into fine crumbs. Spread the crumbs into a shallow 25 cm/10 in diameter dish. Cook, uncovered, on Full for 5–6 minutes, stirring four times, until you can feel in your fingers that the crumbs are dry and crisp. Allow to cool, stirring round from time to time, then store in an airtight container. They will keep almost indefinitely in a cool place.

Nut Burgers

Makes 12

These are by no means new, particularly to vegetarians and vegans, but the combination of nuts gives these burgers an outstanding flavour, and the crunchy texture is equally appetising. They can be served hot with a sauce, cold with salad and mayonnaise, halved horizontally and used as a sandwich filling, or eaten just as they are for a snack.

30 ml/2 tbsp butter or margarine
125 g/4 oz/1 cup unskinned whole almonds
125 g/4 oz/1 cup pecan nut pieces
125 g/4 oz/1 cup cashew nut pieces, toasted
125 g/4 oz/2 cups fresh soft brown breadcrumbs
1 medium onion, grated
2.5 ml/½ tsp salt
5 ml/1 tsp made mustard
30 ml/2 tbsp cold milk

Melt the butter or margarine, uncovered, on Full for 1–1½ minutes. Grind the nuts fairly finely in a blender or food processor. Tip out and combine with the remaining ingredients including the butter or margarine. Divide into 12 equal pieces and shape into ovals. Arrange round the edge of a large greased plate. Cook, uncovered, on Full for 4 minutes, turning once. Allow to stand for 2 minutes.

Nutkin Cake

Serves 6–8

Prepare as for Nut Burgers, but substitute 350 g/12 oz/3 cups ground mixed nuts of your choice for the almonds, pecans and cashews. Shape into a 20 cm/8 in round and put on a greased plate. Cook, uncovered, on Full for 3 minutes. Allow to stand for 5 minutes, then cook on Full for a further 2½ minutes. Allow to stand for 2 minutes. Serve hot or cold, cut into wedges.

Buckwheat

Serves 4

Also known as Saracen corn and native to Russia, buckwheat is related to no other grain. It is the small fruit of a sweetly perfumed pink-flowering plant which is a member of the dock family. The basis of blinis (or Russian pancakes), the grain is a hearty, earthy staple and is a healthy substitute for potatoes with meat and poultry.

175 g/6 oz/1 cup buckwheat
1 egg, beaten
5 ml/1 tsp salt
750 ml/1¼ pts/3 cups boiling water

Mix the buckwheat and egg in a 2 litre/3½ pt/8½ cup dish. Toast, uncovered, on Full for 4 minutes, stirring and breaking up with a fork every minute. Add the salt and water. Stand on a plate in the microwave in case of spillage and cook, uncovered, on Full for 22 minutes, stirring four times. Cover with a plate and allow to stand for 4 minutes. Fork round before serving.

Bulgar

Serves 6–8

Also called burghal, burghul or cracked wheat, this grain is one of the staples of the Middle East. It is now widely available from supermarkets and health food shops.

225 g/8 oz/1¼ cups bulgar
600 ml/1 pt/2½ cups boiling water
5–7.5 ml/1–1½ tsp salt

Put the bulgar in a 1.75 litre/3 pt/7½ cup dish. Toast, uncovered, on Full for 3 minutes, stirring every minute. Stir in the boiling water and salt. Cover with a plate and allow to stand for 6–15 minutes, depending on the variety of bulgar used, until the grain is al dente, like pasta. Fluff up with a fork and eat hot or cold.

Bulgar with Fried Onion

Serves 4

1 onion, grated
15 ml/1 tbsp olive or sunflower
1 quantity Bulgar

Put the onion and oil in a small dish. Cook, uncovered, on Full for 4 minutes, stirring three times. Add to the cooked bulgar at the same time as the water and salt.

Tabbouleh

Serves 4

Coloured deep green by the parsley, this dish evokes the Lebanon and is one of the most appetising salads imaginable, a perfect accompaniment to many dishes from vegetarian nut cutlets to roast lamb. It also makes an attractive starter, arranged over salad greens on individual plates.

1 quantity Bulgar
120–150 ml/4–5 fl oz/½–2/3 cup finely chopped flatleaf parsley
30 ml/2 tbsp chopped mint leaves
1 medium onion, finely grated
15 ml/1 tbsp olive oil
Salt and freshly ground black pepper
Salad leaves
Diced tomatoes, diced cucumber and black olives, to garnish

Cook the bulgar as directed. Transfer half the quantity to a bowl and mix in the parsley, mint, onion, oil and plenty of salt and pepper to taste. When cold, arrange on salad leaves and decorate attractively with the garnish. Use the remaining bulgar in any way you wish.

Sultan's Salad

Serves 4

A personal favourite and, topped with pieces of Feta cheese and served with pitta bread, it makes a complete meal.

1 quantity Bulgar
1–2 garlic cloves, crushed
1 carrot, grated
15 ml/1 tbsp chopped mint leaves
60 ml/4 tbsp chopped parsley
Juice of 1 large lemon, strained
45 ml/3 tbsp olive or sunflower oil, or a mixture of both
Salad greens
Toasted almonds and green olives, to garnish

Cook the bulgar as directed, then stir in the garlic, carrot, mint, parsley, lemon juice and oil. Arrange on a plate lined with salad greens and stud with toasted almonds and green olives.

Couscous

Serves 4

Couscous is both a grain and the name of a North African meat or vegetable stew. Made from durum wheat semolina (cream of wheat), it looks like tiny, perfectly rounded pearls. It used to be hand-made by dedicated and talented home cooks but is now available in packets and can be cooked in a flash, thanks to a French technique that does away with the laborious and slow task of steaming. You can substitute couscous for any of the dishes made with bulgar (pages 209–10).

250 g/9 oz/1½ cups bought couscous
300 ml/½ pt/1¼ cups boiling water
5–10 ml/1–2 tsp salt

Put the couscous in a 1.75 litre/3 pt/7½ cup dish and toast, uncovered, on Full for 3 minutes, stirring every minute. Add the water and salt and fork round. Cover with a plate and cook on Full for 1 minute. Allow to stand in the microwave for 5 minutes. Fluff up with a fork before serving.

Grits

Serves 4

Grits (hominy grits) is a an almost-white North American cereal based on maize (corn). It is eaten with hot milk and sugar or with butter and salt and pepper. It is available from speciality food shops like Harrods in London.

150 g/5 oz/scant 1 cup grits
150 ml/¼ pt/2/3 cup cold water
600 ml/1 pt/2½ cups boiling water
5 ml/1 tsp salt

Put the grits in a 2.5 litre/4½ pt/11 cup bowl. Mix smoothly with the cold water, then stir in the boiling water and salt. Cook, uncovered, on Full for 8 minutes, stirring four times. Cover with a plate and allow to stand for 3 minutes before serving.

Gnocchi alla Romana

Serves 4

Gnocchi is often to be found in Italian restaurants, where it is well liked. It makes a substantial and wholesome lunch or supper dish with salad and uses economical ingredients.

600 ml/1 pt/2½ cups cold milk
150 g/5 oz/¾ cup semolina (cream of wheat)
5 ml/1 tsp salt
50 g/2 oz/¼ cup butter or margarine
75 g/3 oz/¾ cup grated Parmesan cheese
2.5 ml/½ tsp continental made mustard
1.5 ml/¼ tsp grated nutmeg
1 large egg, beaten
Mixed salad
Tomato ketchup (catsup)

Mix half the cold milk smoothly with the semolina in a 1.5 litre/2½ pt/6 cup dish. Heat the remaining milk, uncovered, on Full for 3 minutes. Stir into the semolina with the salt. Cook, uncovered, on Full for 7 minutes until very thick, stirring four or five times to keep the mixture smooth. Remove from the microwave and mix in half the butter, half the cheese and all the mustard, nutmeg and egg. Cook, uncovered, on Full for 1 minute. Cover with a plate and allow to stand for 1 minute. Spread in an oiled or buttered shallow 23 cm/9 in square dish. Cover loosely with kitchen paper and leave in the cool until firm and set. Cut into 2.5 cm/1 in squares. Arrange in a 23 cm/9 in buttered round dish in overlapping rings. Sprinkle with the remaining cheese, dot with flakes of the remaining butter and reheat in a hot oven for 15 minutes until golden brown. Serve very hot with salad and tomato sauce.

Ham Gnocchi

Serves 4

Prepare as for Gnocchi alla Romana, but add 75 g/3 oz/¾ cup chopped Parma ham with the warm milk.

Millet

Serves 4–6

A pleasing and delicate grain, related to sorghum, which is an off-beat substitute for rice. If eaten with pulses (peas, beans and lentils), it makes a well-balanced, protein-rich meal.

175 g/6 oz/1 cup millet
750 ml/1¼ pts/3 cups boiling water or stock
5 ml/1 tsp salt

Put the millet in a 2 litre/3½ pt/8½ cup dish. Toast, uncovered, on Full for 4 minutes, stirring twice. Mix in the water and salt. Stand on a plate in case of spillage. Cook, uncovered, on Full for 20–25 minutes until all the water has been absorbed. Fluff up with a fork and eat straight away.

Polenta

Serves 6

A bright yellow grain made from corn, similar to semolina (cream of wheat) but coarser. It is a staple starch food in Italy and Romania, where it is much respected and often eaten as a side dish with meat, poultry, egg and vegetable dishes. In recent years it has become a trendy restaurant speciality, often cut into squares and served grilled (broiled) or fried (sautéed) with the sauces similar to those used for spaghetti.

150 g/5 oz/¾ cup polenta
5 ml/1 tsp salt
125 ml/¼ pt/2/3 cup cold water
600 ml/1 pt/2½ cups boiling water or stock

Put the polenta and salt in a 2 litre/3½ pt/8½ cup dish. Blend smoothly with the cold water. Gradually mix in the boiling water or stock. Stand on a plate in case of spillage. Cook, uncovered, on Full for 7–8 minutes until very thick, stirring four times. Cover with a plate and allow to stand for 3 minutes before serving.

Grilled Polenta

Serves 6

Prepare as for Polenta. When cooked, spread in a buttered or oiled 23 cm/9 in square dish. Smooth the top with a knife dipped in and out of hot water. Cover loosely with kitchen paper and allow to cool completely. Cut into squares, brush with olive or corn oil and grill (broil) or fry (sauté) conventionally until golden brown.

Polenta with Pesto

Serves 6

Prepare as for Polenta, but add 20 ml/4 tsp red or green pesto with the boiling water.

Polenta with Sun-dried Tomato or Olive Paste

Serves 6

Prepare as for Polenta, but add 45 ml/3 tbsp sun-dried tomato or olive paste with the boiling water.

Quinoa

Serves 2–3

A fairly new-on-the-scene high-protein grain from Peru with a curiously crunchy texture and slightly smoky flavour. It goes with all foods and makes a novel substitute for rice.

125 g/4 oz/2/3 cup quinoa
2.5 ml/½ tsp salt
550 ml/18 fl oz/2 1/3 cups boiling water

Put the quinoa in a 1.75 litre/3 pt/7½ cup bowl. Toast, uncovered, on Full for 3 minutes, stirring once. Add the salt and water and mix in thoroughly. Cook on Full for 15 minutes, stirring four times. Cover and allow to stand for 2 minutes.

Romanian Polenta

Serves 4

Romania's notoriously rich national dish – mamaliga.

1 quantity Polenta
75 g/3 oz/1/3 cup butter
4 freshly poached large eggs
100 g/4 oz/1 cup Feta cheese, crumbled
150 ml/¼ pt/2/3 cup soured (dairy sour) cream

Prepare the polenta and leave in the dish in which it was cooked. Beat in half the butter. Spoon equal mounds on to four warmed plates and make an indentation in each. Fill with the eggs, sprinkle with the cheese and top with the remaining butter and the cream. Eat straight away.

Curried Rice

Serves 4

Suitable as an accompaniment for most oriental and Asiatic foods, especially Indian.

30 ml/2 tbsp groundnut (peanut) oil
2 onions, finely chopped
225 g/8 oz/1 cup basmati rice
2 small bay leaves
2 whole cloves
Seeds from 4 cardamom pods
30–45 ml/2–3 tbsp mild curry powder
5 ml/1 tsp salt
600 ml/1 pt/2½ cups boiling water or vegetable stock

Put the oil in a 2.25 litre/4 pt/10 cup dish. Heat, uncovered, on Full for 1 minute. Mix in the onions. Cook, uncovered, on Full for 5 minutes. Stir in all the remaining ingredients. Cover with clingfilm (plastic wrap) and slit it twice to allow steam to escape. Cook on Full for 15 minutes, turning the dish four times. Allow to stand for 2 minutes. Fork round lightly and serve.

Cottage Cheese and Rice Casserole

Serves 3–4

A great amalgam of tastes and textures brought back from North America some years ago.

225 g/8 oz/1 cup brown rice
50 g/2 oz/¼ cup wild rice
1.25 litre/2¼ pts/5½ cups boiling water
10 ml/2 tsp salt
4 spring onions (scallions), coarsely chopped
1 small green chilli, seeded and chopped
4 tomatoes, blanched, skinned and sliced
125 g/4 oz button mushrooms, sliced
225 g/8 oz/1 cup cottage cheese
75 g/3 oz/¾ cup Cheddar cheese, grated

Put the brown and wild rice in a 2.25 litre/4 pt/10 cup dish. Stir in the water and salt. Cover with clingfilm (plastic wrap) and slit it twice to allow steam to escape. Cook on Full for 40–45 minutes until the rice is plump and tender. Drain, if necessary, and set aside. Fill a 1.75 litre/3 pt/7½ cup casserole dish (Dutch oven) with alternate layers of rice, onions, chilli, tomatoes, mushrooms and cottage cheese. Sprinkle thickly with the grated Cheddar. Cook, uncovered, on Full for 7 minutes, turning the dish twice.

Italian Risotto

Serves 2–3

2.5–5 ml/½–1 tsp saffron powder or 5 ml/1 tsp saffron strands
50 g/2 oz/¼ cup butter
5 ml/1 tsp olive oil
1 large onion, peeled and grated
225 g/8 oz/1 cup easy-cook risotto rice
600 ml/1 pt/2½ cups boiling water or chicken stock
150 ml/¼ pt/2/3 cup dry white wine
5 ml/1 tsp salt
50 g/2 oz/½ cup grated Parmesan cheese

If using saffron strands, crumble them between your fingers into an egg cup of hot water and allow to stand for 10–15 minutes. Put half the butter and the oil in a 1.75 litre/3 pt/7½ cup dish. Heat, uncovered, on Defrost for 1 minute. Stir in the onion. Cook, uncovered, on Full for 5 minutes. Stir in the rice, water or stock and wine and either the saffron strands with the water, or the saffron powder. Cover with clingfilm (plastic wrap) and slit it twice to allow steam to escape. Cook on Full for 14 minutes, turning the dish three times. Gently fork in the remaining butter, followed by the salt and half the Parmesan cheese. Cook, uncovered, on Full for 4–8 minutes, stirring gently with a fork every 2 minutes, until the rice has absorbed all the liquid. The cooking time will depend on the rice used. Spoon into dishes and sprinkle the remaining cheese on top.

Mushroom Risotto

Serves 2–3

Break 20 g/1 oz dried mushrooms, porcini for preference, into smallish pieces, wash thoroughly under cold running water and then soak them for 10 minutes in the boiling water or chicken stock used in the Italian Risotto recipe. Proceed as for Italian Risotto.

Brazilian Rice

Serves 3–4

15 ml/1 tbsp olive or corn oil
30 ml/2 tbsp dried onion
225 g/8 oz/1 cup American long-grain or basmati rice
5–10 ml/1–2 tsp salt
600 ml/1 pt/2½ cups boiling water
2 large tomatoes, blanched, skinned and chopped

Pour the oil in a 2 litre/3½ pt/8½ cup dish. Add the dried onion. Cook, uncovered, on Full for 1¼ minutes. Stir in all the remaining ingredients. Cover with clingfilm (plastic wrap) and slit it twice to allow steam to escape. Cook on Full for 15 minutes, turning the dish four times. Allow to stand for 2 minutes. Fork round lightly and serve.

Spanish Rice

Serves 6

A North American special that has little to do with Spain other than the addition of peppers and tomatoes! Eat with poultry and egg dishes.

225 g/8 oz/1 cup easy-cook long-grain rice
600 ml/1 pt/2½ cups boiling water
10 ml/2 tsp salt
30 ml/2 tbsp corn or sunflower oil
2 onions, finely chopped
1 green (bell) pepper, seeded and coarsely chopped
400 g/14 oz/1 large can chopped tomatoes

Cook the rice in the water with half the salt as directed. Keep hot. Pour the oil into a 1.75 litre/3 pt/7½ cup bowl. Heat, uncovered, on Full for 1 minute. Stir in the onions and pepper. Cook, uncovered, on Full for 5 minutes, stirring twice. Mix in the tomatoes. Heat, uncovered, on Full for 3½ minutes. Fork in the hot rice with the remaining salt and serve straight away.

Plain Turkish Pilaf

Serves 4

225 g/8 oz/1 cup easy-cook risotto rice
Boiling water or vegetable stock
5 ml/1 tsp salt
40 g/1½ oz/3 tbsp butter

Cook the rice in the boiling water or stock with the salt added as directed. Add the butter to the dish or bowl. Allow to stand for 10 minutes. Uncover and fork round. Cover with a plate and reheat on Full for 3 minutes.

Rich Turkish Pilaf

Serves 4

225 g/8 oz/1 cup easy-cook risotto rice
Boiling water
5 ml/1 tsp salt
5 cm/2 in piece cinnamon stick
40 g/1½ oz/3 tbsp butter
15 ml/1 tbsp olive oil
2 onions, finely chopped
60 ml/4 tbsp toasted pine nuts
25 g/1 oz lambs' or chicken liver, cut into small pieces
30 ml/2 tbsp currants or raisins
2 tomatoes, blanched, skinned and chopped

Cook the rice in the water and salt, in a large dish or bowl, as directed with the cinnamon stick added. Set aside. Put the butter and oil in a 1.25 litre/2¼ pt/5½ cup bowl and heat, uncovered, on Full for 1 minute. Mix in all the remaining ingredients. Cover with a plate and cook on Full for 5 minutes, stirring twice. Stir gently into the hot rice with a fork. Cover as before and reheat on Full for 2 minutes.

Thai Rice with Lemon Grass, Lime Leaves and Coconut

Serves 4

A marvel of exquisite delicacy, appropriate for all Thai-style chicken and fish dishes.

250 g/9 oz/generous 1 cup Thai rice
400 ml/14 fl oz/1¾ cups canned coconut milk
2 fresh lime leaves
1 blade lemon grass, split lengthways, or 15 ml/1 tbsp chopped lemon balm leaves
7.5 ml/1½ tsp salt

Tip the rice into a 1.5 litre/2½ pt/6 cup dish. Pour the coconut milk into a measuring jug and make up to 600 ml/1 pt/2½ cups with cold water. Heat, uncovered, on Full for 7 minutes until it begins to bubble and boil. Stir gently into the rice with all the remaining ingredients. Cover with clingfilm (plastic wrap) and slit it twice to allow steam to escape. Cook on Full for 14 minutes. Allow to stand for 5 minutes. Uncover and remove the lemon grass, if used. Fork round gently and eat the slightly soft and sticky rice straight away.

Okra with Cabbage

Serves 6

A curiosity from the Gabon, mild or hot depending on the amount of chilli included.

30 ml/2 tbsp groundnut (peanut) oil
450 g/1 lb Savoy cabbage or spring greens (collard greens), finely shredded
200 g/7 oz okra (ladies' fingers), topped, tailed and cut into chunks
1 onion, grated
300 ml/½ pt/1¼ cups boiling water
10 ml/2 tsp salt
45 ml/3 tbsp pine nuts, lightly toasted under the grill (broiler)
2.5–20 ml/¼–4 tsp chilli powder

Pour the oil into a 2.25 litre/4 pt/10 cup casserole dish (Dutch oven). Stir in the greens and okra followed by the remaining ingredients. Mix well. Cover with clingfilm (plastic wrap) and slit it twice to allow steam to escape. Cook on Full for 7 minutes. Allow to stand for for 5 minutes. Cook on Full for a further 3 minutes. Drain if necessary and serve.

Red Cabbage with Apple

Serves 8

Magnificent with hot gammon, goose and duck, red cabbage is of Scandinavian and North European descent, a sweet-sour and now quite smart side dish, on its best behaviour in the microwave where it stays a deep rosy colour.

900 g/2 lb red cabbage
450 ml/¾ pt/2 cups boiling water
7.5 ml/1½ tsp salt
3 onions, finely chopped
3 cooking (tart) apples, peeled and grated
30 ml/2 tbsp light soft brown sugar
2.5 ml/½ tsp caraway seeds
30 ml/2 tbsp cornflour (cornstarch)
45 ml/3 tbsp malt vinegar
15 ml/1 tbsp cold water

Trim the cabbage, removing any bruised or damaged outer leaves. Cut into quarters and remove the hard central stalk, then shred as finely as possible. Put into a 2.25 litre/4 pt/10 cup dish. Add half the boiling water and 5 ml/1 tsp of the salt. Cover with a plate and cook on Full for 10 minutes, turning the dish four times. Stir well, then mix in the remaining boiling water and remaining salt, the onions, apples, sugar and caraway seeds. Cover with clingfilm (plastic wrap) and slit it twice to allow steam to escape. Cook on Full for 20 minutes, turning the dish four times. Remove from the microwave. Mix the cornflour smoothly with the vinegar and cold water. Add to the hot cabbage and mix well. Cook, uncovered, on Full for 10 minutes, stirring three times. Leave until cold before chilling overnight. To serve, re-cover with fresh clingfilm and slit it twice to allow steam to escape, then heat on Full for 5–6 minutes before serving. Alternatively, transfer portions to side plates and cover each with kitchen paper, then reheat individually on Full for 1 minute each.

Red Cabbage with Wine

Serves 8

Prepare as for Red Cabbage with Apples, but substitute 250 ml/8 fl oz/1 cup red wine for half the boiling water.

Norwegian Sour Cabbage

Serves 8

900 g/2 lb white cabbage
90 ml/6 tbsp water
60 ml/4 tbsp malt vinegar
60 ml/4 tbsp granulated sugar
10 ml/2 tsp caraway seeds
7.5–10 ml/1½–2 tsp salt

Trim the cabbage, removing any bruised or damaged outer leaves. Cut into quarters and remove the hard central stalk, then shred as finely as possible. Put into a 2.25 litre/4 pt/10 cup dish with all the remaining ingredients. Mix thoroughly with two spoons. Cover with clingfilm (plastic wrap) and slit it twice to allow steam to escape. Cook on Defrost for 45 minutes, turning the dish four times. Leave at kitchen temperature overnight for the flavours to mature. To serve, put individual servings on to side plates and cover each with kitchen paper. Reheat individually on Full, allowing about 1 minute each. Securely cover and then refrigerate any leftovers.

Greek-style Stewed Okra with Tomatoes

Serves 6–8

Very marginally Eastern in character, this slightly off-beat vegetable dish has become a viable proposition now that okra (ladies' fingers) is more widely available. This recipe is excellent with lamb or as a dish in its own right, served with rice.

900 g/2 lb okra, topped and tailed
Salt and freshly ground black pepper
90 ml/6 tbsp malt vinegar
45 ml/3 tbsp olive oil
2 onions, peeled and finely chopped
6 tomatoes, blanched, skinned and coarsely chopped
15 ml/1 tbsp light soft brown sugar

Spread out the okra on a large flat plate. To reduce the chances of the okra splitting and taking on a slimy feel, sprinkle with salt and the vinegar. Allow to stand for for 30 minutes. Wash and wipe dry on kitchen paper. Pour the oil into a 2.5 litre/4½ pt/11 cup dish and add the onions. Cook, uncovered, on Full for 7 minutes, stirring three times. Stir in all the remaining ingredients including the okra and season to taste. Cover with a plate and cook on Full for 9–10 minutes, stirring three or four times, until the okra is tender. Allow to stand for 3 minutes before serving.

Greens with Tomatoes, Onions and Peanut Butter

Serves 4–6

Try this Malawi speciality with sliced white bread as a vegetarian main course or serve as a side dish with chicken.

450 g/1 lb spring greens (collard greens), finely shredded
150 ml/¼ pt/2/3 cup boiling water
5–7.5 ml/1–1½ tsp salt
4 tomatoes, blanched, skinned and sliced
1 large onion, finely chopped
60 ml/4 tbsp crunchy peanut butter

Place the greens in a 2.25 litre/4 pt/10 cup dish. Mix in the water and salt. Cover with clingfilm (plastic wrap) and slit it twice to allow steam to escape. Cook on Full for 20 minutes. Uncover and stir in the tomatoes, onion and peanut butter. Cover as before and cook on Full for 5 minutes.

Sweet-sour Creamed Beetroot

Serves 4

This attractive way of presenting beetroot dates back to 1890, but it's currently back in fashion.

450 g/1 lb cooked beetroot (red beets), coarsely grated
150 ml/¼ pt/2/3 cup double (heavy) cream
Salt
15 ml/1 tbsp vinegar
30 ml/2 tbsp demerara sugar

Put the beetroot in a 900 ml/1½ pt/3¾ cup dish with the cream and salt to taste. Cover with a plate and heat through on Full for 3 minutes, stirring once. Stir in the vinegar and sugar and serve straight away.

Beetroot in Orange

Serves 4–6

A lively and original accompaniment to Christmas meats and poultry.

450 g/1 lb cooked beetroot (red beets), peeled and sliced
75 ml/5 tbsp freshly squeezed orange juice
15 ml/1 tbsp malt vinegar
2.5 ml/½ tsp salt
1 garlic clove, peeled and crushed

Place the beetroot in a shallow 18 cm/7 in diameter dish. Beat together the remaining ingredients and pour over the beetroot. Cover with clingfilm (plastic wrap) and slit it twice to allow steam to escape. Cook on Full for 6 minutes, turning the dish three times. Allow to stand for 1 minute.

Scalloped Celeriac

Serves 6

A handsome and gourmet-style winter side dish that teams happily with fish and poultry.

4 lean rashers (slices) bacon, chopped
900 g/2 lb celeriac (celery root)
300 ml/½ pt/1¼ cups cold water
15 ml/1 tbsp lemon juice
7.5 ml/1½ tsp salt
300 ml/½ pt/1¼ cups single (light) cream
1 small bag potato crisps (chips), crushed in the bag

Put the bacon on a plate and cover with kitchen paper. Cook on Full for 3 minutes. Peel the celeriac thickly, wash well and cut each head into eight pieces. Place in a 2.25 litre/4 pt/10 cup dish with the water, lemon juice and salt. Cover with clingfilm (plastic wrap) and slit it twice to allow steam to escape. Cook on Full for 20 minutes, turning the dish four times. Drain. Slice the celeriac and return to the dish. Stir in the bacon and cream and sprinkle with the crisps. Cook, uncovered, on Full for 4 minutes, turning the dish twice. Allow to stand for 5 minutes before serving.

Celeriac with Orange Hollandaise Sauce

Serves 6

Celeriac with a gloriously golden, gleaming topping of citrus Hollandaise sauce to try with duck and game.

900 g/2 lb celeriac (celery root)
300 ml/½ pt/1¼ cups cold water
15 ml/1 tbsp lemon juice
7.5 ml/1½ tsp salt
Maltese Sauce
1 very sweet orange, peeled and segmented

Peel the celeriac thickly, wash well and cut each head into eight pieces. Place in a 2.25 litre/4 pt/10 cup dish with the water, lemon juice and salt. Cover with clingfilm (plastic wrap) and slit it twice to allow steam to escape. Cook on Full for 20 minutes, turning the dish four times. Drain. Slice the celeriac and return to the dish. Keep hot. Make the Maltese Sauce and spoon over the celeriac. Garnish with the orange segments.

Slimmers' Vegetable Pot

Serves 2

Prepare as for Slimmer's Fish Pot but omit the fish. Add the diced flesh of 2 avocados to the cooked vegetables with the spices and herbs. Cover and reheat on Full for 1½ minutes.

Slimmers' Vegetable Pot with Eggs

Serves 2

Prepare as for Slimmer's Vegetable Pot, but sprinkle each portion with 1 chopped hard-boiled (hard-cooked) egg.

Ratatouille

Serves 6–8

An explosion of Mediterranean flavours and colours is part and parcel of this glorious vegetable pot-pourri. Hot, cold or warm – it seems to go with everything.

60 ml/4 tbsp olive oil
3 onions, peeled and coarsely chopped
1–3 garlic cloves, crushed
225 g/8 oz courgettes (zucchini), thinly sliced
350 g/12 oz/3 cups cubed aubergine (eggplant)
1 large red or green (bell) pepper, seeded and chopped
3 ripe tomatoes, skinned, blanched and chopped
30 ml/2 tbsp tomato purée (paste)
20 ml/4 tsp light soft brown sugar
10 ml/2 tsp salt
45–60 ml/3–4 tbsp chopped parsley

Pour the oil into a 2.5 litre/4½ pt/11 cup dish. Heat, uncovered, on Full for 1 minute. Mix in the onions and garlic. Cook, uncovered, on Full for 4 minutes. Stir in all the remaining ingredients except half the parsley. Cover with a plate and cook on Full for 20 minutes, stirring three or four times. Uncover and cook on Full for 8–10 minutes, stirring four times, until most of the liquid has evaporated. Mix in the remaining parsley. Serve straight away or cool, cover and chill if to be eaten later.

Caramelised Parsnips

Serves 4

Ideal with all poultry and beef roasts, choose baby parsnips no bigger than large carrots for this.

450 g/1 lb small parsnips, thinly sliced
45 ml/3 tbsp water
25 g/1 oz/2 tbsp butter
7.5 ml/1½ tbsp dark soft brown sugar
Salt

Put the parsnips in a 1.25 litre/2¼ pt/5½ cup dish with the water. Cover with clingfilm (plastic wrap) and slit it twice to allow steam to escape. Cook on Full for 8–10 minutes, turning the dish and gently shaking the contents twice, until tender. Drain off the water. Add the butter and sugar and toss the parsnips to coat them thoroughly. Heat, uncovered, on Full for 1–1½ minutes until glazed. Sprinkle with salt and eat straight away.

Parsnips with Egg and Butter Crumb Sauce

Serves 4

450 g/1 lb parsnips, diced
45 ml/3 tbsp water
75 g/3 oz/1/3 cup unsalted (sweet) butter
4 spring onions (scallions), finely chopped
45 ml/3 tbsp light-coloured toasted breadcrumbs
1 hard-boiled (hard-cooked) egg, grated
30 ml/2 tbsp finely chopped parsley
Juice of ½ small lemon

Place the parsnips in a 1.5 litre/2½ pt/6 cup dish with the water. Cover with clingfilm (plastic wrap) and slit it twice to allow steam to escape. Cook on Full for 8–10 minutes. Allow to stand while preparing the sauce. Put the butter in a measuring jug and melt, uncovered, on Defrost for 2–2½ minutes. Stir in the onions and cook, uncovered, on Defrost for 3 minutes, stirring twice. Mix in all the remaining ingredients and heat on Defrost for 30 seconds. Drain the parsnips and transfer to a warmed serving dish. Coat with the crumb sauce and serve straight away.

Broccoli with Cheese Supreme

Serves 4–6

450 g/1 lb broccoli
60 ml/4 tbsp water
5 ml/1 tsp salt
150 ml/¼ pt/2/3 cup soured (dairy sour) cream
125 g/4 oz/1 cup Cheddar or Jarlsberg cheese, grated
1 egg
5 ml/1 tsp mild made mustard
2.5 ml/½ tsp paprika
1.5 ml/¼ tsp grated nutmeg

Wash the broccoli, separate into small florets and put into a deep 20 cm/8 in diameter dish with the water and salt. Cover with clingfilm (plastic wrap) and slit it twice to allow steam to escape. Cook on Full for 12 minutes. Drain thoroughly. Beat together the remaining ingredients and spoon over the broccoli. Cover with a plate and cook on Full for 3 minutes. Allow to stand for 2 minutes.

Guvetch

Serves 6–8

A vibrantly coloured and flavour-packed Bulgarian relation of ratatouille. Serve on its own with rice, pasta or polenta or as an accompaniment to egg, meat and poultry dishes.

450 g/1 lb French or Kenya (green) beans, topped and tailed
4 onions, very thinly sliced
3 garlic cloves, crushed
60 ml/4 tbsp olive oil
6 (bell) peppers in mixed colours, seeded and cut into strips
6 tomatoes, blanched, skinned and chopped
1 green chilli, seeded and finely chopped (optional)
10–15 ml/2–3 tsp salt
15 ml/1 tbsp caster (superfine) sugar

Cut each bean into three pieces. Put the onions and garlic in a 2.5 litre/4½ pt/11 cup dish with the oil. Stir well to mix. Cook, uncovered, on Full for 4 minutes. Thoroughly mix in all the remaining ingredients including the beans. Cover with a plate and cook on Full for 20 minutes, stirring three times. Uncover and cook on Full for a further 8–10 minutes, stirring four times, until most of the liquid has evaporated. Serve straight away or cool, cover and chill if to be eaten later.

Celery Cheese with Bacon

Serves 4

6 rashers (slices) streaky bacon
350 g/12 oz celery, diced
30 ml/2 tbsp boiling water
30 ml/2 tbsp butter or margarine
30 ml/2 tbsp plain (all-purpose) flour
300 ml/½ pt/1¼ cups warm full-cream milk
5 ml/1 tsp English made mustard
225 g/8 oz/2 cups Cheddar cheese, grated
Salt and freshly ground black pepper
Paprika
Fried (sautéed) bread, to serve

Put the bacon on a plate and cover with kitchen paper. Cook on Full for 4–4½ minutes, turning the plate once. Drain off the fat, then coarsely chop the bacon. Put the celery in a separate dish with the boiling water. Cover with a plate and cook on Full for 10 minutes, turning the dish twice. Drain and reserve the liquid. Put the butter in a 1.5 litre/2½ pt/6 cup dish. Melt, uncovered, on Defrost for 1–1½ minutes. Stir in the flour and cook on Full for 1 minute. Gradually blend in the milk. Cook, uncovered, on Full for 4–5 minutes until smoothly thickened, whisking every minute. Mix in the celery water, celery, bacon, mustard and two-thirds of the cheese. Season to taste. Transfer the mixture to a clean dish. Sprinkle the remaining cheese on top and dust with paprika. Reheat, uncovered, on Full for 2 minutes. Serve with fried bread.

Artichoke Cheese with Bacon

Serves 4

Prepare as for Celery Cheese with Bacon, but omit the celery. Put 350 g/12 oz Jerusalem artichokes in a bowl with 15 ml/1 tbsp lemon juice and 90 ml/6 tbsp boiling water. Cover with clingfilm (plastic wrap) and slit it twice to allow steam to escape. Cook on Full for 12–14 minutes until tender. Drain, reserving 45 ml/3 tbsp of the water. Add the artichokes and the water to the sauce with the mustard, bacon and cheese.

Karelian Potatoes

Serves 4

A recipe from eastern Finland for springtime potatoes.

450 g/1 lb new potatoes, washed but unpeeled
30 ml/2 tbsp boiling water
125 g/4 oz/½ cup butter, at kitchen temperature
2 hard-boiled (hard-cooked) eggs, chopped

Put the potatoes in a 900 ml/1½ pt/3¾ cup dish with the boiling water. Cover with a plate and cook on Full for 11 minutes, stirring twice. Meanwhile, beat the butter to a smooth cream and stir in the eggs. Drain the potatoes and stir in the egg mixture while the potatoes are still very hot. Serve straight away.

Dutch Potato and Gouda Casserole with Tomatoes

Serves 4

A filling and warming vegetarian casserole that can be served with cooked green vegetables or a crunchy salad.

750 g/1½ lb cooked potatoes, thickly sliced
3 large tomatoes, blanched, skinned and thinly sliced
1 large red onion, coarsely grated
30 ml/2 tbsp finely chopped parsley
175 g/6 oz/1½ cups Gouda cheese, grated
Salt and freshly ground black pepper
30 ml/2 tbsp cornflour (cornstarch)
30 ml/2 tbsp cold milk
150 ml/¼ pt/2/3 cup hot water or vegetable stock
Paprika

Fill a buttered 1.5 litre/2½ pt/6 cup dish with alternate layers of potatoes, tomatoes, onion, parsley and two-thirds of the cheese, sprinkling salt and pepper between the layers. Mix the cornflour smoothly with the cold milk, then gradually whisk in the hot water or stock. Pour down the side of the dish. Sprinkle the remaining cheese on top and dust with paprika. Cover with kitchen paper and heat through on Full for 12–15 minutes. Allow to stand for 5 minutes before serving.

Buttered and Fluffed Sweet Potatoes with Cream

Serves 4

450 g/1 lb sweet pink-skinned and yellow-fleshed potatoes (not yams),
peeled and diced
60 ml/4 tbsp boiling water
45 ml/3 tbsp butter or margarine
60 ml/4 tbsp whipped cream, warmed
Salt and freshly ground black pepper

Put the potatoes in a 1.25 litre/2¼ pt/5½ cup dish. Add the water. Cover with clingfilm (plastic wrap) and slit it twice to allow steam to escape. Cook on Full for 10 minutes, turning the dish three times. Allow to stand for 3 minutes. Drain and finely mash. Thoroughly beat in the butter and cream. Season well to taste. Transfer to a serving dish, cover with a plate and reheat on Full for 1½ –2 minutes.

Maître d'Hôtel Sweet Potatoes

Serves 4

450 g/1 lb sweet pink-skinned and yellow-fleshed potatoes (not yams), peeled and diced

60 ml/4 tbsp boiling water

45 ml/3 tbsp butter or margarine

45 ml/3 tbsp chopped parsley

Put the potatoes in a 1.25 litre/2¼ pt/5½ cup dish. Add the water. Cover with clingfilm (plastic wrap) and slit it twice to allow steam to escape. Cook on Full for 10 minutes, turning the dish three times. Allow to stand for 3 minutes, then drain. Add the butter and toss to coat the potatoes, then sprinkle with the parsley.

Creamed Potatoes

Serves 4–6

Potatoes cooked in the microwave retain their flavour and colour and have an excellent texture. Their nutrients are conserved because the amount of water used for cooking is minimal. Fuel is saved and there is no pan to wash – you can even cook the potatoes in their own serving dish. Peel potatoes as thinly as possible to retain the vitamins.

900 g/2 lb peeled potatoes, cut into chunks

90 ml/6 tbsp boiling water

30–60 ml/2–4 tbsp butter or margarine

90 ml/6 tbsp warm milk

Salt and freshly ground black pepper

Put the potato chunks in a 1.75 litre/3 pt/7½ cup with the water. Cover with clingfilm (plastic wrap) and slit it twice to allow steam to escape. Cook on Full for 15–16 minutes, turning the dish four times, until tender. Drain if necessary, then mash finely, beating in the butter or margarine and milk alternately. Season. When light and fluffy, rough up with a fork and reheat, uncovered, on Full for 2–2½ minutes.

Creamed Potatoes with Parsley

Serves 4–6

Prepare as for Creamed Potatoes, but mix in 45–60 ml/3–4 tbsp chopped parsley with the seasoning. Reheat for an extra 30 seconds.

Creamed Potatoes with Cheese

Serves 4–6

Prepare as for Creamed Potatoes, but mix in 125 g/4 oz/1 cup grated hard cheese with the seasoning. Reheat for an extra 1½ minutes.

Hungarian Potatoes with Paprika

Serves 4

50 g/2 oz/¼ cup margarine or lard
1 large onion, finely chopped
750 g/1½ lb potatoes, cut into small chunks
45 ml/3 tbsp dried pepper flakes
10 ml/2 tsp paprika
5 ml/1 tsp salt
300 ml/½ pt/1¼ cups boiling water
60 ml/4 tbsp soured (dairy sour) cream

Put the margarine or lard in a 1.75 litre/3 pt/7½ cup dish. Heat, uncovered, on Full for 2 minutes until sizzling. Add the onion. Cook, uncovered, on Full for 2 minutes. Stir in the potatoes, pepper flakes, paprika, salt and boiling water. Cover with clingfilm (plastic wrap) and slit it twice to allow steam to escape. Cook on Full for 20 minutes, turning the dish four times. Allow to stand for 5 minutes. Spoon out on to warmed plates and top each with 15 ml/1 tbsp soured cream.

Dauphine Potatoes

Serves 6

Gratin dauphinoise – one of the French greats and an experience to be relished. Serve with a leafy salad or baked tomatoes, or as an accompaniment to meat, poultry, fish and eggs.

900 g/2 lb waxy potatoes, very thinly sliced
1–2 garlic cloves, crushed
75 ml/5 tbsp melted butter or margarine
175 g/6 oz/1½ cups Emmental or Gruyère (Swiss) cheese
Salt and freshly ground black pepper
300 ml/½ pt/1¼ cups full-cream milk
Paprika

To tenderise the potatoes, place in a large bowl and cover with boiling water. Leave for 10 minutes, then drain. Combine the garlic with the butter or margarine. Butter a deep 25 cm/10 in diameter dish. Beginning and ending with potatoes, fill the dish with alternate layers of potato slices, two-thirds of the cheese and two-thirds of the butter mixture, sprinkling salt and pepper between the layers. Pour the milk carefully down the side of the dish, then scatter over the remaining cheese and garlic butter. Sprinkle with paprika. Cover with clingfilm (plastic wrap) and slit it twice to allow steam to escape. Cook on Full for 20 minutes, turning the dish four times. The potatoes should be slightly al dente, like pasta, but if you would prefer them softer, cook on Full for an extra 3–5 minutes. Allow to stand for 5 minutes, then uncover and serve.

Savoyard Potatoes

Serves 6

Prepare as for Dauphine Potatoes, but substitute stock, or half white wine and half stock, for the milk.

Château Potatoes

Serves 6

Prepare as for Dauphine Potatoes, but substitute medium cider for the milk.

Potatoes with Almond Butter Sauce

Serves 4–5

450 g/1 lb new potatoes, unpeeled and scrubbed
30 ml/2 tbsp water
75 g/3 oz/1/3 cup unsalted (sweet) butter
75 g/3 oz/¾ cup flaked (slivered) almonds, toasted and crumbled
15 ml/1 tbsp fresh lime juice

Place the potatoes in a 1.5 litre/2½ pt/6 cup dish with the water. Cover with clingfilm (plastic wrap) and slit it twice to allow steam to escape. Cook on Full for 11–12 minutes until tender. Allow to stand while preparing the sauce. Put the butter in a measuring jug and melt, uncovered, on Defrost for 2–2½ minutes. Stir in the remaining ingredients. Toss with the drained potatoes and serve.

Mustard and Lime Tomatoes

Serves 4

A fresh zestiness makes the tomatoes attractive as a dish on the side with lamb and poultry, and also with salmon and mackerel.

4 large tomatoes, halved horizontally
Salt and freshly ground black pepper
5 ml/1 tsp finely grated lime peel
30 ml/2 tbsp wholegrain mustard
Juice of 1 lime

Stand the tomatoes, in a circle, cut sides up, round the edge of a large plate. Sprinkle with salt and pepper. Thoroughly combine the remaining ingredients and spread over the tomatoes. Cook, uncovered, on Full for 6 minutes, turning the plate three times. Allow to stand for 1 minute.

Braised Cucumber

Serves 4

1 cucumber, peeled
30 ml/2 tbsp butter or margarine, at kitchen temperature
2.5–5 ml/½–1 tsp salt
30 ml/2 tbsp finely chopped parsley or coriander (cilantro) leaves

Slice the cucumber very thinly, leave to stand for 30 minutes, then wring dry in a clean tea towel (dish cloth). Put the butter or margarine in a 1.25 litre/2¼ pt/5½ cup dish and melt, uncovered, on Defrost for 1–1½ minutes. Stir in the cucumber and salt, tossing gently until well coated with butter. Cover with a plate and cook on Full for 6 minutes, stirring twice. Uncover and stir in the parsley or coriander.

Braised Cucumber with Pernod

Serves 4

Prepare as for Braised Cucumber, but add 15 ml/1 tbsp Pernod with the cucumber.

Marrow Espagnole

Serves 4

A summer side dish to complement poultry and fish.

15 ml/1 tbsp olive oil
1 large onion, peeled and chopped
3 large tomatoes, blanched, skinned and chopped
450 g/1 lb marrow (squash), peeled and cubed
15 ml/1 tbsp marjoram or oregano, chopped
5 ml/1 tsp salt
Freshly ground black pepper

Heat the oil in a 1.75 litre/3 pt/7½ cup dish, uncovered, on Full for 1 minute. Stir in the onion and tomatoes. Cover with a plate and cook on Full for 3 minutes. Mix in all remaining ingredients, adding pepper to taste. Cover with a plate and cook on Full for 8–9 minutes until the marrow is tender. Allow to stand for 3 minutes.

Gratin of Courgettes and Tomatoes

Serves 4

3 tomatoes, blanched, skinned and coarsely chopped
4 courgettes (zucchini), topped, tailed and thinly sliced
1 onion, chopped
15 ml/1 tbsp malt or rice vinegar
30 ml/2 tbsp chopped flatleaf parsley
1 garlic clove, crushed
Salt and freshly ground black pepper
75 ml/5 tbsp Cheddar or Emmental cheese, grated

Put the tomatoes, courgettes, onion, vinegar, parsley and garlic in a deep 20 cm/8 in diameter dish. Season to taste and toss well to mix. Cover with clingfilm (plastic wrap) and slit it twice to allow steam to escape. Cook on Full for 15 minutes, turning the dish three times. Uncover and sprinkle with the cheese. Either brown conventionally under the grill (broiler) or, to save time, return to the microwave and heat on Full for 1–2 minutes until the cheese bubbles and melts.

Courgettes with Juniper Berries

Serves 4–5

8 juniper berries
30 ml/2 tbsp butter or margarine
450 g/1 lb courgettes (zucchini), topped, tailed and thinly sliced
2.5 ml/½ tsp salt
30 ml/2 tbsp finely chopped parsley

Crush the juniper berries lightly with the back of a wooden spoon. Put the butter or margarine in a deep 20 cm/8 in diameter dish. Melt, uncovered, on Defrost for 1–1½ minutes. Mix in the juniper berries, courgettes and salt and spread in an even layer to cover the base of the dish. Cover with clingfilm (plastic wrap) and slit it twice to allow steam to escape. Cook on Full for 10 minutes, turning the dish four times. Allow to stand for 2 minutes. Uncover and sprinkle with the parsley.

Buttered Chinese Leaves with Pernod

Serves 4

A cross in texture and flavour between white cabbage and firm lettuce, Chinese leaves make a highly presentable cooked vegetable and are greatly enhanced by the addition of Pernod, which adds a delicate and subtle hint of aniseed.

675 g/1½ lb Chinese leaves, shredded
50 g/2 oz/¼ cup butter or margarine
15 ml/1 tbsp Pernod
2.5–5 ml/½–1 tsp salt

Put the shredded leaves in a 2 litre/3½ pt/8½ cup dish. In a separate dish, melt the butter or margarine on Defrost for 2 minutes. Add to the cabbage with the Pernod and salt and toss gently to mix. Cover with a plate and cook on Full for 12 minutes, stirring twice. Allow to stand for 5 minutes before serving.

Chinese-style Bean Sprouts

Serves 4

450 g/1 lb fresh bean sprouts
10 ml/2 tsp dark soy sauce
5 ml/1 tsp Worcestershire sauce
5 ml/1 tsp onion salt

Toss all the ingredients together in a large mixing bowl. Transfer to a deep 20 cm/8 in diameter casserole dish (Dutch oven). Cover with a plate and cook on Full for 5 minutes. Allow to stand for 2 minutes, then stir round and serve.

Carrots with Orange

Serves 4–6

50 g/2 oz/¼ cup butter or margarine
450 g/1 lb carrots, grated
1 onion, grated
15 ml/1 tbsp fresh orange juice
5 ml/1 tsp finely grated orange peel
5 ml/1 tsp salt

Put the butter or margarine in a deep 20 cm/8 in diameter dish. Melt, uncovered, on Defrost for 1½ minutes. Stir in all the remaining ingredients and mix thoroughly. Cover with clingfilm (plastic wrap) and slit it twice to allow steam to escape. Cook on Full for 15 minutes, turning the dish twice. Allow to stand for 2–3 minutes before serving.

Braised Chicory

Serves 4

An unusual vegetable side dish that tastes faintly of asparagus. Serve with egg and poultry dishes.

4 heads chicory (Belgian endive)
30 ml/2 tbsp butter or margarine
1 vegetable stock cube
15 ml/1 tbsp boiling water
2.5 ml/½ tsp onion salt
30 ml/2 tbsp lemon juice

Trim the chicory, discarding any bruised or damaged outer leaves. Remove a cone-shaped core from the base of each to reduce bitterness. Cut the chicory into 1.5 cm/½ in thick slices and put in a 1.25 litre/2¼ pt/5½ cup casserole dish (Dutch oven). Melt the butter or margarine separately on Defrost for 1½ minutes. Pour over the chicory. Crumble the stock cube into the boiling water, then add the salt and lemon juice. Spoon over the chicory. Cover with clingfilm (plastic wrap) and slit it twice to allow steam to escape. Cook on Full for 9 minutes, turning the dish three times. Allow to stand for 1 minute before serving with the juices from the dish.

Braised Carrots with Lime

Serves 4

An intensely orange-coloured carrot dish, designed for meat stews and game.

450 g/1 lb carrots, thinly sliced
60 ml/4 tbsp boling water
30 ml/2 tbsp butter
1.5 ml/¼ tsp turmeric
5 ml/1 tsp finely grated lime peel

Place the carrots in a 1.25 litre/2¼ pt/5½ cup dish with the boiling water. Cover with clingfilm (plastic wrap) and slit it twice to allow steam to escape. Cook on Full for 9 minutes, turning the dish three times. Allow to stand for 2 minutes. Drain. Immediately toss in the butter, turmeric and lime peel. Eat straight away.

Fennel in Sherry

Serves 4

900 g/2 lb fennel
50 g/2 oz/¼ cup butter or margarine
2.5 ml/½ tsp salt
7.5 ml/1½ tsp French mustard
30 ml/2 tbsp medium-dry sherry
2.5 ml/½ tsp dried or 5 ml/1 tsp chopped fresh tarragon

Wash and dry the fennel. Discard any brown areas but leave on the 'fingers' and green fronds. Melt the butter or margarine, uncovered, on Defrost for 1½–2 minutes. Gently beat in the remaining ingredients. Quarter each head of fennel and place in a deep 25 cm/10 in diameter dish. Coat with the butter mixture. Cover with a plate and cook on Full for 20 minutes, turning the dish four times. Allow to stand for 7 minutes before serving.

Wine-braised Leeks with Ham

Serves 4

5 narrow leeks, about 450g/1 lb in all
30 ml/2 tbsp butter or margarine, at kitchen temperature
225 g/8 oz/2 cups cooked ham, chopped
60 ml/4 tbsp red wine
Salt and freshly ground black pepper

Trim off the whiskery ends of the leeks, then cut off all but 10 cm/4 in of green 'skirt' from each. Carefully halve the leeks lengthways almost to the top. Wash thoroughly between the leaves under cold running water to remove any earth or grit. Put the butter or margarine in a 25 x 20 cm/10 x 8 in dish. Melt on Defrost for 1–1½ minutes, then brush over the base and sides. Arrange the leeks, in a single layer, over the base. Sprinkle with the ham and wine and season. Cover with clingfilm (plastic wrap) and slit it twice to allow steam to escape. Cook on Full for 15 minutes, turning the dish twice. Allow to stand for 5 minutes.

Casseroled Leeks

Serves 4

5 narrow leeks, about 450g/1 lb in all
30 ml/2 tbsp butter or margarine
60 ml/4 tbsp vegetable stock
Salt and freshly ground black pepper

Trim off the whiskery ends of the leeks, then cut off all but 10 cm/4 in of green 'skirt' from each. Carefully halve the leeks lengthways almost to the top. Wash thoroughly between the leaves under cold running water to remove any earth or grit. Cut into 1.5 cm/½ in thick slices. Place in a 1.75 litre/3 pt/7½ cup casserole dish (Dutch oven). In a separate bowl, melt the butter or margarine on Defrost for 1½ minutes. Add the stock and season well to taste. Spoon over the leeks. Cover with a plate and cook on Full for 10 minutes, stirring twice.

Casseroled Celery

Serves 4

Prepare as for Casseroled Leeks, but substitute 450 g/1 lb washed celery for the leeks. If liked, add a small chopped onion and cook for an extra 1½ minutes.

Meat-stuffed Peppers

Serves 4

4 green (bell) peppers
30 ml/2 tbsp butter or margarine
1 onion, finely chopped
225 g/8 oz/2 cups lean minced (ground) beef
30 ml/2 tbsp long-grain rice
5 ml/1 tsp dried mixed herbs
5 ml/1 tsp salt
120 ml/4 fl oz/¼ cup hot water

Cut the tops off the peppers and reserve. Discard the inside fibres and seeds from each pepper. Cut a thin sliver off each base so that they stand upright without toppling over. Put the butter or margarine in a dish and heat on Full for 1 minute. Add the onion. Cook, uncovered, on Full for 3 minutes. Mix in the meat, breaking it up with a fork. Cook, uncovered, on Full for 3 minutes. Stir in the rice, herbs, salt and 60 ml/4 tbsp of the water. Spoon the mixture into the peppers. Arrange upright and close together in a clean deep dish. Replace the lids and pour the rest of the water into the dish around the peppers for gravy. Cover with clingfilm (plastic wrap) and slit it twice to allow steam to escape. Cook on Full for 15 minutes, turning the dish twice. Allow to stand for 10 minutes before serving.

Meat-stuffed Peppers with Tomato

Serves 4

Prepare as for Meat-stuffed Peppers, but substitute tomato juice sweetened with 10 ml/2 tsp caster (superfine) sugar for the water.

Turkey-stuffed Peppers with Lemon and Thyme

Serves 4

Prepare as for Meat-stuffed Peppers, but substitute minced (ground) turkey for the beef and 2.5 ml/½ tsp thyme for the mixed herbs. Add 5 ml/1 tsp finely grated lemon peel.

Polish-style Creamed Mushrooms

Serves 6

Commonplace in Poland and Russia where mushrooms take pride of place on any table. Eat with new potatoes and boiled eggs.

30 ml/2 tbsp butter or margarine
450 g/1 lb button mushrooms
30 ml/2 tbsp cornflour (cornstarch)
30 ml/2 tbsp cold water
300 ml/½ pt/1¼ cups soured (dairy sour) cream
10 ml/2 tsp salt

Put the butter or margarine in a deep 2.25 litre/4 pt/10 cup dish. Melt, uncovered, on Defrost for 1½ minutes. Mix in the mushrooms. Cover with a plate and cook on Full for 5 minutes, stirring twice. Blend the cornflour smoothly with the water and stir in the cream. Gently stir into the mushrooms. Cover as before and cook on Full for 7–8 minutes, stirring three times, until thick and creamy. Fold in the salt and eat straight away.

Paprika Mushrooms

serves 6

Prepare as for Polish-style Creamed Mushrooms, but add 1 crushed garlic clove to the butter or margarine before melting. Mix in 15 ml/1 tbsp each tomato purée (paste) and paprika with the mushrooms. Serve with small pasta.

Curried Mushrooms

serves 6

Prepare as for Polish-style Creamed Mushrooms, but add 15–30 ml/1–2 tbsp mild curry paste and one crushed garlic clove to the butter or margarine before melting. Substitute thick plain yoghurt for the cream and fold in 10 ml/2 tsp caster (superfine) sugar with the salt. Serve with rice.

Lentil Dhal

Serves 6–7

Distinctively Oriental with its roots in India, this Lentil Dhal is graciously flavoured with a myriad spices and can be served either as an accompaniment to curries or by itself with rice as a nutritious and complete meal.

50 g/2 oz/¼ cup ghee, butter or margarine
4 onions, chopped
1–2 garlic cloves, crushed
225 g/8 oz/1 1/3 cups orange lentils, thoroughly rinsed
5 ml/1 tsp turmeric
5 ml/1 tsp paprika
2.5 ml/½ tsp ground ginger
20 ml/4 tsp garam masala
1.5 ml/¼ tsp cayenne pepper
Seeds from 4 green cardamom pods
15 ml/1 tbsp tomato purée (paste)
750 ml/1¼ pts/3 cups boiling water
7.5 ml/1½ tsp salt
Chopped coriander (cilantro) leaves, to garnish

Put the ghee, butter or margarine in a 1.75 litre/3 pt/7½ cup casserole dish (Dutch oven). Heat, uncovered, on Full for 1 minute. Mix in the onions and garlic. Cover with a plate and cook on Full for 3 minutes. Stir in all the remaining ingredients Cover with a plate and cook on Full for 15 minutes, stirring four times. Allow to stand for 3 minutes. If too thick for personal taste, thin down with a little extra boiling water. Fluff up with fork before serving garnished with the coriander.

Dhal with Onions and Tomatoes

Serves 6–7

3 onions
50 g/2 oz/¼ cup ghee, butter or margarine
1–2 garlic cloves, crushed
225 g/8 oz/1 1/3 cups orange lentils, thoroughly rinsed
3 tomatoes, blanched, skinned and chopped
5 ml/1 tsp turmeric
5 ml/1 tsp paprika
2.5 ml/½ tsp ground ginger
20 ml/4 tsp garam masala
1.5 ml/¼ tsp cayenne pepper
Seeds from 4 green cardamom pods
15 ml/1 tbsp tomato purée (paste)
750 ml/1¼ pts/3 cups boiling water
7.5 ml/1½ tsp salt
1 large onion, thinly sliced
10 ml/2 tsp sunflower or corn oil

Thinly slice 1 onion and chop the remainder. Put the ghee, butter or margarine in a 1.75 litre/3 pt/7½ cup casserole dish (Dutch oven). Heat, uncovered, on Full for 1 minute. Mix in the chopped onions and garlic. Cover with a plate and cook on Full for 3 minutes. Stir in all the remaining ingredients. Cover with a plate and cook on Full for 15 minutes, stirring four times. Allow to stand for 3 minutes. If too thick for personal taste, thin down with a little extra boiling water. Separate the sliced onion into rings and fry (sauté) conventionally in the oil until lightly golden and crisp. Fluff up the dhal with a fork before serving garnished with the onion rings. (Alternatively, omit the sliced onion and instead garnish with ready-prepared fried onions available from supermarkets.)

Vegetable Madras

Serves 4

25 g/1 oz/2 tbsp ghee or 15 ml/1 tbsp groundnut (peanut) oil
1 onion, peeled and chopped
1 leek, trimmed and chopped
2 garlic cloves, crushed
15 ml/1 tbsp hot curry powder
5 ml/1 tsp ground cumin
5 ml/1 tsp garam masala
2.5 ml/½ tsp turmeric
Juice of 1 small lemon
150 ml/¼ pt/⅔ cup vegetable stock
30 ml/2 tbsp tomato purée (paste)
30 ml/2 tbsp toasted cashew nuts
450 g/1 lb mixed cooked root vegetables, diced
175 g/6 oz/¾ cup brown rice, boiled
Popadoms, to serve

Put the ghee or oil in a 2.5 litre/4½ pt/11 cup dish. Heat, uncovered, on Full for 1 minute. Add the onion, leek and garlic and mix in thoroughly. Cook, uncovered, on Full for 3 minutes. Add the curry powder, cumin, garam masala, turmeric and lemon juice. Cook, uncovered, on Full for 3 minutes, stirring twice. Add the stock, tomato purée and cashew nuts. Cover with an inverted plate and cook on Full for 5 minutes. Stir in the vegetables. Cover as before and heat through on Full for 4 minutes. Serve with the brown rice and popadoms.

Mixed Vegetable Curry

Serves 6

1.6 kg/3½ lb mixed vegetables, such as red or green (bell) peppers; courgettes (zucchini); unpeeled aubergines (eggplants); carrots; potatoes; Brussels sprouts or broccoli; onions; leeks

30 ml/2 tbsp groundnut (peanut) or corn oil

2 garlic cloves, crushed

60 ml/4 tbsp tomato purée (paste)

45 ml/3 tbsp garam masala

30 ml/2 tbsp mild, medium or hot curry powder

5 ml/1 tsp ground coriander (cilantro)

5 ml/1 tsp ground cumin

15 ml/1 tbsp salt

1 large bay leaf

400 g/14 oz/1 large can chopped tomatoes

15 ml/1 tbsp caster (superfine) sugar

150 ml/¼ pt/2/3 cup boiling water

250 g/9 oz/generous 1 cup basmati or long-grain rice, boiled

Thick plain yoghurt, to serve

Prepare all the vegetables according to type. Cut into small cubes or slice where appropriate. Place in a 2.75 litre/5 pt/12 cup deep dish. Mix in all the remaining ingredients except the boiling water and rice. Cover with a large plate and cook on Full for 25–30 minutes, stirring four times, until the vegetables are tender but still firm to the bite. Remove the bay leaf, blend in the water and adjust the seasonings to taste – the curry may need some extra salt. Serve with the rice and a bowl of thick plain yoghurt.

Jellied Mediterranean Salad

Serves 6

300 ml/½ pt/1¼ cups cold vegetable stock or vegetable cooking water

15 ml/1 tbsp powdered gelatine

45 ml/3 tbsp tomato juice

45 ml/3 tbsp red wine

1 green (bell) pepper, seeded and cut into strips

2 tomatoes, blanched, skinned and chopped

30 ml/2 tbsp drained capers

50g /2 oz/¼ cup chopped gherkins (cornichons)

12 stuffed olives, sliced

10 ml/2 tsp anchovy sauce

Pour 45 ml/3 tbsp of the stock or vegetable cooking water in a bowl. Stir in the gelatine. Allow to stand for 5 minutes to soften. Melt, uncovered, on Defrost for 2–2½ minutes. Stir in the remaining stock with the tomato juice and wine. Cover when cold, then chill until just beginning to thicken and set. Place the pepper strips in a bowl and cover with boiling water. Leave for 5 minutes to soften, then drain. Stir the tomatoes and pepper strips into the setting jelly with all the remaining ingredients. Transfer to a 1.25 litre/2¼ pt/5½ cup wetted jelly mould or basin. Cover and chill for several hours until firm. To serve, dip the mould or basin in and out of bowl of hot water to loosen, then run a hot wet knife gently round the sides. Invert on to a wetted plate before serving. (The wetting stops the jelly sticking.)

Jellied Greek Salad

Serves 6

Prepare as for Jellied Mediterranean Salad, but omit the capers and gherkins (cornichons). Add 125 g/4 oz/1 cup finely diced Feta cheese and 1 small chopped onion. Substitute stoned (pitted) black olives for stuffed.

Jellied Russian Salad

Serves 6

Prepare as for Jellied Mediterranean Salad, but substitute 90 ml/6 tbsp mayonnaise for the tomato juice and wine and 225 g/8 oz/2 cups diced carrots and potatoes for the tomatoes and (bell) pepper. Add 30 ml/2 tbsp cooked peas.

Kohlrabi Salad with Mustardy Mayonnaise

Serves 6

900 g/2 lb kohlrabi
75 ml/5 tbsp boiling water
5 ml/1 tsp salt
10 ml/2 tsp lemon juice
60–120 ml/4–6 tbsp thick mayonnaise
10–20 ml/2–4 tsp wholegrain mustard
Sliced radishes, to garnish

Peel the kohlrabi thickly, wash well and cut each head into eight pieces Place in a 1.25 litre/3 pt/7½ cup dish with the water, salt and lemon juice. Cover with clingfilm (plastic wrap) and slit it twice to allow steam to escape. Cook on Full for 10–15 minutes, turning the dish three times, until tender. Drain and slice or dice and put in a mixing bowl. Mix together the mayonnaise and mustard and toss the kohlrabi in this mixture until the pieces are thoroughly coated. Transfer to a serving dish and garnish with the radish slices.

Beetroot, Celery and Apple Cups

Serves 6

60 ml/4 tbsp cold water
15 ml/1 tbsp powdered gelatine
225 ml/8 fl oz/1 cup apple juice
30 ml/2 tbsp raspberry vinegar
5 ml/1 tsp salt
225 g/8 oz cooked (not pickled) beetroot (red beets), coarsely grated
1 eating (dessert) apple, peeled and coarsely grated
1 celery stalk, cut into thin matchsticks
1 small onion, chopped

Pour 45 ml/3 tbsp of the cold water in a small bowl and stir in the gelatine. Leave to stand for 5 minutes to soften. Melt, uncovered, on Defrost for 2–2½ minutes. Stir in the remaining cold water with the apple juice, vinegar and salt. Cover when cold, then chill until just beginning to thicken and set. Add the beetroot, apple, celery and onion to the part-set jelly and stir gently until thoroughly combined. Transfer to six small wetted cups, then cover and chill until firm and set. Turn out on to individual plates.

Mock Waldorf Cups

Serves 6

Prepare as for Beetroot, Celery and Apple Cups, but add 30 ml/2 tbsp chopped walnuts with the vegetables and apple.

Celeriac Salad with Garlic, Mayonnaise and Pistachios

Serves 6

900 g/2 lb celeriac (celery root)
300 ml/½ pt/1¼ cups cold water
15 ml/1 tbsp lemon juice
7.5 ml/1½ tsp salt
1 garlic clove, crushed
45 ml/3 tbsp coarsely chopped pistachio nuts
60–120 ml/4–8 tbsp thick mayonnaise
Radicchio leaves and whole pistachio nuts, to garnish

Peel the celeriac thickly, wash well and cut each head into eight pieces. Place in a 2.25 litre/4 pt/10 cup dish with the water, lemon juice and salt. Cover with clingfilm (plastic wrap) and slit it twice to allow steam to escape. Cook on Full for 20 minutes, turning the dish four times. Drain and slice and put in a mixing bowl. Add the garlic and chopped pistachio nuts. While still warm, toss with the mayonnaise until the pieces of celeriac are thoroughly coated. Transfer to a serving dish. Garnish with radicchio leaves and pistachios before serving, if possible while still slightly warm.

Continental Celeriac Salad

Serves 4

An assembly of fine and complementary flavours makes this a suitable Christmas salad to go with cold turkey and gammon.

750 g/1½ lb celeriac (celery root)
75 ml/5 tbsp boiling water
5 ml/1 tsp salt
10 ml/2 tsp lemon juice
For the dressing:
30 ml/2 tbsp corn or sunflower oil
15 ml/1 tbsp malt or cider vinegar
15 ml/1 tbsp made mustard
2.5–5 ml/½–1 tsp caraway seeds
1.5 ml/¼ tsp tsp salt
5 ml/1 tsp caster (superfine) sugar
Freshly ground black pepper

Peel the celeriac thickly and cut it into small cubes. Place in a 1.75 litre/3 pt/7½ cup dish. Add the boiling water, salt and lemon juice. Cover with clingfilm (plastic wrap) and slit it twice to allow steam to escape. Cook on Full for 10–15 minutes, turning the dish three times, until tender. Drain. Thoroughly beat together all the remaining ingredients. Add to the hot celeriac and toss thoroughly. Cover and allow to cool. Serve at room temperature.

Celeriac Salad with Bacon

Serves 4

Prepare as for Continental Celeriac Salad, but add 4 rashers (slices) bacon, crisply grilled (broiled) and crumbled, at the same time as the dressing.

Artichoke Salad with Peppers and Eggs in Warm Dressing

Serves 6

400 g/14 oz/1 large can artichoke hearts, drained
400 g/14 oz/1 large can red pimientos, drained
10 ml/2 tsp red wine vinegar
60 ml/4 tbsp lemon juice
125 ml/4 fl oz/½ cup olive oil
1 garlic clove, crushed
5 ml/1 tsp continental mustard
5 ml/1 tsp salt
5 ml/1 tsp caster (superfine) sugar
4 large hard-boiled (hard-cooked) eggs, shelled and grated
225 g/8 oz/2 cups Feta cheese, diced

Halve the artichokes and cut the pimientos into strips. Arrange alternately round a large plate, leaving a hollow in the centre. Put the vinegar, lemon juice, oil, garlic, mustard, salt and sugar in small bowl. Heat, uncovered, on Full for 1 minute, beating twice. Pile the eggs and cheese in a mound in the centre of the salad and gently spoon over the warm dresssing.

Sage and Onion Stuffing

Makes 225–275 g/8–10 oz/1 1/3–1 2/3 cups

For pork.

25 g/1 oz/2 tbsp butter or margarine
2 onions, pre-boiled (see table page 45), chopped
125 g/4 oz/2 cups white or brown breadcrumbs
5 ml/1 tsp dried sage
A little water or milk
Salt and freshly ground black pepper

Put the butter or margarine in a 1 litre/1¾ pt/4¼ cup dish. Heat, uncovered, on Full for 1 minute. Stir in the onions. Cook, uncovered, on Full for 3 minutes, stirring every minute. Mix in the breadcrumbs and sage and sufficient water or milk to bind to a crumbly consistency. Season to taste. Use when cold.

Celery and Pesto Stuffing

Makes 225–275 g/8–10 oz/1 1/3–1 2/3 cups

For fish and poultry.

Prepare as for Sage and Onion Stuffing, but substitute 2 finely chopped celery stalks for the onions. Before seasoning, stir in 10 ml/2 tsp green pesto.

Leek and Tomato Stuffing

Makes 225–275 g/8–10 oz/1 1/3–1 2/3 cups

For meat and poultry.

25 g/1 oz/2 tbsp butter or margarine
2 leeks, white part only, cut into very thin slices
2 tomatoes, blanched, skinned and chopped
125 g/4 oz/2 cups fresh white breadcrumbs
Salt and freshly ground black pepper
Chicken stock, if necessary

Put the butter or margarine in a 1 litre/1¾ pt/4¼ cup dish. Heat, uncovered, on Full for 1 minute. Stir in the leeks. Cook, uncovered, on Full for 3 minutes, stirring three times. Mix in the tomatoes and breadcrumbs and season to taste. Bind with stock if necessary. Use when cold.

Bacon Stuffing

Makes 225–275 g/8–10 oz/1 1/3–12/3 cups

For meat, poultry and strong-tasting fish.

4 rashers (slices) streaky bacon, chopped into small pieces
25 g/1 oz/2 tbsp butter, margarine or lard
125 g/4 oz/2 cups fresh white breadcrumbs
5 ml/1 tsp Worcestershire sauce
5 ml/1 tsp made mustard
2.5 ml/½ tsp dried mixed herbs
Salt and freshly ground black pepper
Milk, if necessary

Put the bacon in a 1 litre/1¾ pt/4¼ cup dish with the butter, margarine or lard. Cook, uncovered, on Full for 2 minutes, stirring once. Mix in the breadcrumbs, Worcestershire sauce, mustard and herbs and season to taste. Bind with milk if necessary.

Bacon and Apricot Stuffing

Makes 225–275 g/8–10 oz/1 1/3–1 2/3 cups

For poultry and game

Prepare as for Bacon Stuffing, but add 6 well-washed and coarsely chopped apricot halves with the herbs.

Mushroom, Lemon and Thyme Stuffing

Makes 225–275 g/8–10 oz/1 1/3–1 2/3 cups

For poultry.

25 g/1 oz/2 tbsp butter or margarine
125 g/4 oz button mushrooms, sliced
5 ml/1 tsp finely grated lemon peel
2.5 ml/½ tsp dried thyme
1 garlic clove, crushed
125 g/4 oz/2 cups fresh white breadcrumbs
Salt and freshly ground black pepper
Milk, if necessary

Put the butter or margarine in a 1 litre/1¾ pt/4¼ cup dish. Heat, uncovered, on Full for 1 minute. Stir in the mushrooms. Cook, uncovered, on Full for 3 minutes, stirring twice. Mix in the lemon peel, thyme, garlic and breadcrumbs and season to taste. Bind with milk only if the stuffing remains on the dry side. Use when cold.

Mushroom and Leek Stuffing

Makes 225–275 g/8–10 oz/1 1/3–1 2/3 cups

For poultry, vegetables and fish.

25 g/1 oz/2 tbsp butter or margarine
1 leek, white part only, very thinly sliced
125 g/4 oz mushrooms, sliced
125 g/4 oz/2 cups fresh brown breadcrumbs
30 ml/2 tbsp chopped parsley
Salt and freshly ground black pepper
Milk, if necessary

Put the butter or margarine in a 1.25 litre/2¼ pt/5½ cup dish. Heat, uncovered, on Full for 1 minute. Stir in the leek. Cook, uncovered, on Full for 2 minutes, stirring once. Mix in the mushrooms. Cook, uncovered, on Full for 2 minutes, stirring twice. Mix in the breadcrumbs and parsley and season to taste. Bind with milk only if the stuffing remains on the dry side. Use when cold.

Ham and Pineapple Stuffing

Makes 225–275 g/8–10 oz/1 1/3–1 2/3 cups

For poultry.

25 g/1 oz/2 tbsp butter or margarine
1 onion, finely chopped
1 fresh pineapple ring, skin removed and flesh chopped
75 g/3 oz/¾ cup cooked ham, chopped
125 g/4 oz/2 cups fresh white breadcrumbs
Salt and freshly ground black pepper

Put the butter or margarine in a 1 litre/1¾ pt/4¼ cup dish. Heat, uncovered, on Full for 1 minute. Stir in the onion. Cook, uncovered, on Full for 2 minutes, stirring once. Mix in the pineapple and ham. Cook, uncovered, on Full for 2 minutes, stirring twice. Fork in the breadcrumbs and season to taste. Use when cold.

Asian Mushroom and Cashew Nut Stuffing

Makes 225–275 g/8–10 oz/1 1/3–1 2/3 cups

For poultry and fish.

25 g/1 oz/2 tbsp butter or margarine
6 spring onions (scallions), chopped
125 g/4 oz mushrooms, sliced
125 g/4 oz/2 cups fresh brown breadcrumbs
45 ml/3 tbsp cashew nuts, toasted
30 ml/2 tbsp coriander (cilantro) leaves
Salt and freshly ground black pepper
Soy sauce, if necessary

Put the butter or margarine in a 1.25 litre/2¼ pt/5½ cup dish. Heat, uncovered, on Full for 1 minute. Stir in the onions. Cook, uncovered, on Full for 2 minutes, stirring once. Mix in the mushrooms. Cook, uncovered, on Full for 2 minutes, stirring twice. Mix in the breadcrumbs, cashew nuts and coriander and season to taste. Bind with soy sauce only if the stuffing remains on the dry side. Use when cold.

Ham and Carrot Stuffing

Makes 225–275 g/8–10 oz/1 1/3–1 2/3 cups

For poultry, lamb and game.

Prepare as for Ham and Pineapple Stuffing, but substitute 2 grated carrots for the pineapple.

Ham, Banana and Sweetcorn Stuffing

Makes 225–275 g/8–10 oz/1 1/3–1 2/3 cups

For poultry.

Prepare as for Ham and Pineapple Stuffing, but substitute 1 small coarsely mashed banana for the pineapple. Add 30 ml/2 tbsp sweetcorn (corn) with the breadcrumbs.

Italian Stuffing

Makes 225–275 g/8–10 oz/1 1/3–1 2/3 cups

For lamb, poultry and fish.

30 ml/2 tbsp olive oil
1 garlic clove
1 celery stalk, finely chopped
2 tomatoes, blanched, skinned and coarsely chopped
12 stoned (pitted) black olives, halved
10 ml/2 tsp chopped basil leaves
125 g/4 oz/2 cups fresh crumbs made from Italian bread such as ciabatta
Salt and freshly ground black pepper

Put the olive oil in a 1 litre/1¾ pt/4¼ cup dish. Heat, uncovered, on Full for 1 minute. Stir in the garlic and celery. Cook, uncovered, on Full for 2½ minutes, stirring once. Mix in all the remaining ingredients. Use when cold.

Spanish Stuffing

Makes 225–275 g/8–10 oz/1 1/3–1 2/3 cups

For strong fish and poultry.

Prepare as for Italian Stuffing, but substitute halved stuffed olives for the stoned (pitted) black olives. Use ordinary white breadcrumbs instead of crumbs from Italian bread and add 30 ml/2 tbsp flaked (slivered) and toasted almonds.

Orange and Coriander Stuffing

Makes 175 G/6 Oz/1 cup

For meat and poultry.

25 g/1 oz/2 tbsp butter or margarine
1 small onion, finely chopped
125 g/4 oz/2 cups fresh white breadcrumbs
Finely grated peel and juice of 1 orange
45 ml/3 tbsp finely chopped coriander (cilantro) leaves
Salt and freshly ground black pepper
Milk, if necessary

Put the butter or margarine in a 1 litre/1¾ pt/4¼ cup dish. Heat, uncovered, on Full for 1 minute. Stir in the onion. Cook, uncovered, on Full for 3 minutes, stirring once. Mix in the crumbs, orange peel and juice and the coriander (cilantro) and season to taste. Bind with milk only if the stuffing remains on the dry side. Use when cold.

Lime and Coriander Stuffing

Makes 175 g/6 oz/1 cup

For fish.

Prepare as for Orange and Coriander Stuffing, but substitute the grated peel and juice of 1 lime for the orange.

Orange and Apricot Stuffing

Makes 275 g/10 oz/12/3 cups

For rich meats and poultry.

125 g/4 oz dried apricots, washed
Warm black tea
25 g/1 oz/2 tbsp butter or margarine
1 small onion, chopped
5 ml/1 tsp finely grated orange peel
Juice of 1 orange
125 g/4 oz/2 cups fresh white breadcrumbs
Salt and freshly ground black pepper

Soak the apricots in warm tea for at least 2 hours. Drain and snip into small pieces with scissors. Put the butter or margarine in a 1.25 litre/2¼ pt/5½ cup dish. Heat, uncovered, on Full for 1 minute. Add the onion. Cook, uncovered, on Full for 2 minutes, stirring once. Mix in all the remaining ingredients including the apricots. Use when cold.

Apple, Raisin and Walnut Stuffing

Makes 275 g/10 oz/1 2/3 cups

For pork, lamb, duck and goose.

25 g/1 oz/2 tbsp butter or margarine
1 eating (dessert) apple, peeled, quartered, cored and chopped
1 small onion, chopped
30 ml/2 tbsp raisins
30 ml/2 tbsp chopped walnuts
5 ml/1 tsp caster (superfine) sugar
125 g/4 oz/2 cups fresh white breadcrumbs
Salt and freshly ground black pepper

Put the butter or margarine in a 1.25 litre/2¼ pt/5½ cup dish. Heat, uncovered, on Full for 1 minute. Stir in the apple and onion. Cook, uncovered, on Full for 2 minutes, stirring once. Mix in all the remaining ingredients. Use when cold.

Apple, Prune and Brazil Nut Stuffing

Makes 275 g/10 oz/1 2/3 cups

For lamb and turkey.

Prepare as for Apple, Raisin and Walnut Stuffing, but substitute 8 stoned (pitted) and chopped prunes for the raisins and 30 ml/2 tbsp thinly sliced Brazil nuts for the walnuts.

Apple, Date and Hazelnut Stuffing

Makes 275 g/10 oz/1 2/3 cups

For lamb and game.

Prepare as for Apple, Raisin and Walnut Stuffing, but substitute 45 ml/3 tbsp chopped dates for the raisins and 30 ml/2 tbsp toasted and chopped hazelnuts for the walnuts.

Garlic, Rosemary and Lemon Stuffing

Makes 175 g/6 oz/1 cup

For lamb and pork.

25 g/1 oz/2 tbsp butter or margarine
2 garlic cloves, crushed
Grated peel of 1 small lemon
5 ml/1 tsp dried rosemary, crushed
15 ml/1 tbsp chopped parsley
125 g/4 oz/2 cups fresh white or brown breadcrumbs
Salt and freshly ground black pepper
Milk or dry red wine, if necessary

Put the butter or margarine in a 1 litre/1¾ pt/4¼ cup dish. Heat, uncovered, on Full for 1 minute. Stir in the garlic and lemon peel. Heat, uncovered, on Full for 30 seconds. Mix round and stir in the rosemary, parsley and breadcrumbs. Season to taste. Bind with milk or wine only if the stuffing remains on the dry side. Use when cold.

Garlic, Rosemary and Lemon Stuffing with Parmesan Cheese

Makes 175 g/6 oz/1 cup.

For beef.

Prepare as for Garlic, Rosemary and Lemon Stuffing, but add 45 ml/3 tbsp grated Parmesan cheese with the breadcrumbs.

Seafood Stuffing

Makes 275 g/10 oz/12/3 cups

For fish and vegetables.

25 g/1 oz/2 tbsp butter or margarine
125 g/4 oz/1 cup whole peeled prawns (shrimp)
5 ml/1 tsp finely grated lemon peel
125 g/4 oz/2 cups fresh white breadcrumbs
1 egg, beaten
Salt and freshly ground black pepper
Milk, if necessary

Put the butter or margarine in a 1 litre/1¾ pt/4¼ cup dish. Heat, uncovered, on Full for 1 minute. Stir in the prawns, lemon peel, breadcrumbs and egg and season to taste. Bind with milk only if the stuffing remains on the dry side. Use when cold.

Parma Ham Stuffing

Makes 275 g/10 oz/1 2/3 cups

For poultry.

Prepare as for Seafood Stuffing, but substitute 75 g/3 oz/¾ cup coarsely chopped Parma ham for the prawns (shrimp).

Sausagemeat Stuffing

Makes 275 g/10 oz/1 2/3 cups

For poultry and pork.

25 g/1 oz/2 tbsp butter or margarine
225 g/8 oz/1 cup pork or beef sausagemeat
1 small onion, grated
30 ml/2 tbsp finely chopped parsley
2.5 ml/½ tsp mustard powder
1 egg, beaten

Put the butter or margarine in a 1 litre/1¾ pt/4¼ cup dish. Heat, uncovered, on Full for 1 minute. Mix in the sausagemeat and onion. Cook, uncovered, on Full for 4 minutes, stirring every minute to ensure the sausagemeat is thoroughly broken up. Mix in all the remaining ingredients. Use when cold.

Sausagemeat and Liver Stuffing

Makes 275 g/10 oz/1 2/3 cups

For poultry.

Prepare as for Sausagemeat Stuffing, but reduce the sausagemeat to 175 g/6 oz/¾ cup. Add 50 g/2 oz/½ cup coarsely chopped chicken livers with the sausagemeat and onion.

Sausagemeat and Sweetcorn Stuffing

Makes 275 g/10 oz/1 2/3 cups

For poultry.

Prepare as for Sausagemeat Stuffing, but stir in 30–45 ml/2–3 tbsp cooked sweetcorn (corn) at the end of the cooking time.

Sausagemeat and Orange Stuffing

Makes 275 g/10 oz/1 2/3 cups

For poultry.

Prepare as for Sausagemeat Stuffing, but add 5–10 ml/1–2 tsp finely grated orange peel at the end of the cooking time

Chestnut Stuffing with Egg

Makes 350 g/12 oz/2 cups

For poultry.

125 g/4 oz/1 cup dried chestnuts, soaked overnight in water, then drained
25 g/1 oz/2 tbsp butter or margarine
1 small onion, grated
1.5 ml/¼ tsp ground nutmeg
125 g/4 oz/2 cups fresh brown breadcrumbs
5 ml/1 tsp salt
1 large egg, beaten
15 ml/1 tbsp double (heavy) cream

Put the chestnuts in a 1.25 litre/2¼ pt/5½ cup casserole dish (Dutch oven) and cover with boiling water. Allow to stand for 5 minutes. Cover with clingfilm (plastic wrap) and slit it twice to allow steam to escape. Cook on Full for 30 minutes until the chestnuts are tender. Drain and allow to cool. Break up into small pieces. Put the butter or margarine in a 1.25 litre/2¼ pt/5½ cup dish. Heat, uncovered, on Full for 1 minute. Add the onion. Cook, uncovered, on Full for 2 minutes, stirring once. Mix in the chestnuts, nutmeg, breadcrumbs, salt and egg. Bind together with the cream. Use when cold.

Chestnut and Cranberry Stuffing

Makes 350 g/12 oz/2 cups

For poultry.

Prepare as for Chestnut Stuffing with Egg, but instead of egg, bind the stuffing with 30–45 ml/2–3 tbsp cranberry sauce. Add a little cream if the stuffing remains on the dry side.

Creamy Chestnut Stuffing

Makes 900 g/2 lb/5 cups

For poultry and fish.

50 g/2 oz/¼ cup butter, margarine or bacon dripping
1 onion, grated
500 g/1lb 2 oz/2¼ cups canned unsweetened chestnut purée
225 g/8 oz/4 cups fresh white breadcrumbs
Salt and freshly ground black pepper
2 eggs, beaten
Milk, if necessary

Put the butter, margarine or dripping in a 1¾ litre/3 pt/7½ cup dish. Heat, uncovered, on Full for 1½ minutes. Add the onion. Cook, uncovered, on Full for 2 minutes, stirring once. Thoroughly mix in the chestnut purée, breadcrumbs, salt and pepper to taste, and the eggs. Bind with milk only if the stuffing remains on the dry side. Use when cold.

Creamy Chestnut and Sausagement Stuffing

Makes 900 g/2 lb/5 cups

For poultry and game.

Prepare as for Creamy Chestnut Stuffing, but substitute 250 g/9 oz/generous 1 cup sausagemeat for half the chestnut purée.

Creamy Chestnut Stuffing with Whole Chestnuts

Makes 900 g/2 lb/5 cups

For poultry.

Prepare as for Creamy Chestnut Stuffing, but add 12 cooked and broken up chestnuts with the breadcrumbs.

Chestnut Stuffing with Parsley and Thyme

Makes 675 g/1½ lb/4 cups

For turkey and chicken.

15 ml/1 tbsp butter or margarine
5 ml/1 tsp sunflower oil
1 small onion, finely chopped
1 garlic clove, crushed
50 g/2 oz/1 cup parsley and thyme dry stuffing mix
440 g/15½ oz/2 cups canned unsweetened chestnut purée
150 ml/¼ pt/2/3 cup hot water
Finely grated peel of 1 lemon
1.5–2.5 ml/¼–½ tsp salt

Put the butter or margarine and oil in a 1.25 litre/2¼ pt/5½ cup bowl. Heat, uncovered, on Full for 25 seconds. Add the onion and garlic. Cook, uncovered, on Full for 3 minutes. Add the dry stuffing mix and stir in well. Cook, uncovered, on Full for 2 minutes, stirring twice. Remove from the microwave. Gradually stir in the chestnut purée alternately with the hot water until smoothly combined. Stir in the lemon peel and salt to taste. Use when cold.

Chestnut Stuffing with Gammon

Makes 675 g/1½ lb/4 cups

For turkey and chicken.

Prepare as for Chestnut Stuffing with Parsley and Thyme, but add 75 g/3 oz/¾ cup chopped gammon with the lemon peel and salt.

Chicken Liver Stuffing

Makes 350 g/12 oz/2 cups

For poultry and game.

125 g/4 oz/2/3 cup chicken livers
25 g/1 oz/2 tbsp butter or margarine
1 onion, grated
30 ml/2 tbsp finely chopped parsley
1.5 ml/¼ tsp ground allspice
125 g/4 oz/2 cups fresh white or brown breadcrumbs
Salt and freshly ground black pepper
Chicken stock, if necessary

Wash the livers and dry on kitchen paper. Cut into small pieces. Put the butter or margarine in a 1.25 litre/2¼ pt/5½ cup dish. Heat, uncovered, on Full for 1 minute. Add the onion. Cook, uncovered, on Full for 2 minutes, stirring once. Add the livers. Cook, uncovered, on Defrost for 3 minutes, stirring 3 times. Mix in the parsley, allspice and breadcrumbs and season to taste. Bind with a little stock only if the stuffing remains on the dry side. Use when cold.

Chicken Liver Stuffing with Pecans and Orange

Makes 350 g/12 oz/2 cups

For poultry and game.

Prepare as for Chicken Liver Stuffing, but add 30 ml/2 tbsp broken pecan nuts and 5 ml/1 tsp finely grated orange peel with the breadcrumbs.

Triple Nut Stuffing

Makes 350 g/12 oz/2 cups

For poultry and meat.

15 ml/1 tbsp sesame oil
1 garlic clove, crushed
125 g/4 oz/2/3 cup finely ground hazelnuts
125 g/4 oz/2/3 cup finely ground walnuts
125 g/4 oz/2/3 cup finely ground almonds
Salt and freshly ground black pepper
1 egg, beaten

Pour the oil into a fairly large dish. Heat, uncovered, on Full for 1 minute. Add the garlic. Cook, uncovered, on Full for 1 minute. Stir in all the nuts and season to taste. Bind with the egg. Use when cold.

Potato and Turkey Liver Stuffing

Makes 675 g/1½ lb/4 cups

For poultry.

450 g/1 lb floury potatoes
25 g/1 oz/2 tbsp butter or margarine
1 onion, chopped
2 rashers (slices) streaky bacon, chopped
5 ml/1 tsp dried mixed herbs
45 ml/3 tbsp finely chopped parsley
2.5 ml/½ tsp ground cinnamon
2.5 ml/½ tsp ground ginger
1 egg, beaten
Salt and freshly ground black pepper

Cook the potatoes as directed for Creamed Potatoes, but using only 60 ml/4 tbsp water. Drain and mash. Put the butter or margarine in a 1.25 litre/2¼ pt/5½ cup dish. Heat, uncovered, on Full for 1 minute. Stir in the onion and bacon. Cook, uncovered, on Full for 3 minutes, stirring twice. Mix in all the remaining ingredients including the potatoes, seasoning to taste. Use when cold.

Rice Stuffing with Herbs

Makes 450 g/1 lb/2 2/3 cups

For poultry.

125 g/4 oz/2/3 cup easy-cook long-grain rice
250 ml/8 fl oz/1 cup boiling water
2.5 ml/½ tsp salt
25 g/1 oz/2 tbsp butter or margarine
1 small onion, grated
5 ml/1 tsp chopped parsley
5 ml/1 tsp coriander (cilantro) leaves
5 ml/1 tsp sage
5 ml/1 tsp basil leaves

Cook the rice with the water and salt as directed. Put the butter or margarine in a 1.25 litre/2¼ pt/5½ cup dish. Heat, uncovered, on Full for 1 minute. Stir in the onion. Cook, uncovered, on Full for 1 minute, stirring once. Mix in the rice and herbs. Use when cold.

Spanish Rice Stuffing with Tomato

Makes 450 g/1 lb/2 2/3 cups

For poultry.

125 g/4 oz/2/3 cup easy-cook long-grain rice
250 ml/8 fl oz/1 cup boiling water
2.5 ml/½ tsp salt
25 g/1 oz/2 tbsp butter or margarine
1 small onion, grated
30 ml/2 tbsp chopped green (bell) pepper
1 tomato, chopped
30 ml/2 tbsp chopped stuffed olives

Cook the rice with the water and salt as directed. Put the butter or margarine in a 1.25 litre/2¼ pt/5½ cup dish. Heat, uncovered, on Full for 1 minute. Stir in the onion, green pepper, tomato and olives. Cook, uncovered, on Full for 2 minute, stirring once. Mix in the rice. Use when cold.

Fruited Rice Stuffing

Makes 450 g/1 lb/2 2/3 cups

For poultry.

125 g/4 oz/2/3 cup easy-cook long-grain rice
250 ml/8 fl oz/1 cup boiling water
2.5 ml/½ tsp salt
25 g/1 oz/2 tbsp butter or margarine
1 small onion, grated
5 ml/1 tsp chopped parsley
6 dried apricot halves, chopped
6 stoned (pitted) prunes, chopped
5 ml/1 tsp finely grated clementine or satsuma peel

Cook the rice with the water and salt as directed. Put the butter or margarine in a 1.25 litre/2¼ pt/5½ cup dish. Heat, uncovered, on Full for 1 minute. Stir in the onion, parsley, apricots, prunes and peel. Cook, uncovered, on Full for 1 minute, stirring once. Mix in the rice. Use when cold.

Far East Rice Stuffing

Makes 450 g/1 lb/2 2/3 cups

For poultry.

Prepare as for Rice Stuffing with Herbs, but use only the coriander (cilantro). Add 6 canned and sliced water chestnuts and 30 ml/2 tbsp coarsely chopped toasted cashew nuts with the onion.

Savoury Rice Stuffing with Nuts

Makes 450 g/1 lb/2 2/3 cups

For poultry.

Prepare as for Rice Stuffing with Herbs, but use only the parsley. Add 30 ml/2 tbsp flaked (slivered) and toasted almonds and 30 ml/2 tbsp salted peanuts with the onion.

Chocolate Crispies

Makes 16

75 g/3 oz/2/3 cup butter or margarine
30 ml/2 tbsp golden (light corn) syrup, melted
15 ml/1 tbsp cocoa (unsweetened chocolate) powder, sifted
45 ml/3 tbsp caster (superfine) sugar
75 g/3 oz/1½ cups cornflakes

Melt the butter or margarine and syrup, uncovered, on Defrost for 2–3 minutes. Stir in the cocoa and sugar. Fold in the cornflakes with a large metal spoon, tossing until well coated. Spoon into paper cake cases (cupcake papers), stand on a board or tray and chill until set.

Devil's Food Cake

Serves 8

A dream of a North American food processor cake, with a light and fluffy texture and deep chocolatey flavour.

100 g/4 oz/1 cup plain (semi-sweet) chocolate, broken into pieces
225 g/8 oz/2 cups self-raising (self-rising) flour
25 g/1 oz/2 tbsp cocoa (unsweetened chocolate) powder
1.5 ml/¼ tsp bicarbonate of soda (baking soda)
200 g/7 oz/scant 1 cup dark soft brown sugar
150 g/5 oz/2/3 cup butter or soft margarine, at kitchen temperature
5 ml/1 tsp vanilla essence (extract)
2 large eggs, at kitchen temperature
120 ml/4 fl oz/½ cup buttermilk or 60 ml/4 tbsp each skimmed milk and plain yoghurt
Icing (confectioners') sugar, for dusting

Closely line the base and sides of a straight-sided deep 20 cm/8 in diameter soufflé dish with clingfilm (plastic wrap). Melt the chocolate in a small bowl on Defrost for 3–4 minutes, stirring twice. Sift the flour, cocoa and bicarbonate of soda directly into a food processor bowl. Add the melted chocolate with all the remaining ingredients and process for about 1 minute or until the ingredients are well combined and the mixture resembles a thick batter. Spoon into the prepared dish and cover loosely with kitchen paper. Cook on Full for 9–10 minutes, turning the dish twice, until the cake has risen to the rim of the dish and the top is covered with small, broken bubbles and looks fairly dry. If any sticky patches remain, cook on Full for a further 20–30 seconds. Allow to stand in the microwave for about 15 minutes (the cake will fall slightly), then take it out and leave to cool until just warm. Carefully lift out of dish by holding the clingfilm and transfer to a wire rack to cool completely. Peel away the clingfilm and dust the top with sifted icing sugar before serving. Store in an airtight container.

Mocha Torte

Serves 8

Prepare as for Devil's Food Cake, but when cold cut the cake horizontally into three layers. Beat 450 ml/¾ pt/2 cups double (heavy) or whipping cream until thick. Sweeten to taste with a little sifted icing (confectioners') sugar, then flavour quite strongly with cold black coffee. Use some of the cream to sandwich the cake layers together, then swirl the remainder over the top and sides. Chill lightly before serving.

Multi-layer Cake

Serves 8

Prepare as for Devil's Food Cake, but when cold cut the cake horizontally into three layers. Sandwich together with apricot jam, whipped cream and grated chocolate or chocolate spread.

Black Forest Cherry Torte

Serves 8

Prepare as for Devil's Food Cake, but when cold cut the cake horizontally into three layers and moisten each with cherry liqueur. Sandwich together with cherry jam (conserve) or cherry fruit filling. Beat 300 ml/½ pt/1¼ cups double (heavy) or whipping cream until thick. Spread over the top and sides of the cake. Press a crushed chocolate flake bar or grated chocolate against the sides, then decorate the top with halved glacé (candied) cherries.

Chocolate Orange Gateau

Serves 8

Prepare as for Devil's Food Cake, but when cold cut the cake horizontally into three layers and moisten each with orange liqueur. Sandwich together with fine-shred orange marmalade and a thin round of marzipan (almond paste). Beat 300 ml/½ pt/1¼ cups double (heavy) or whipping cream until thick. Colour and sweeten lightly with 10–15 ml/2–3 tsp black treacle (molasses), then stir in 10 ml/2 tsp grated orange peel. Spread over the top and sides of the cake.

Chocolate Butter Cream Layer Cake

Serves 8–10

30 ml/2 tbsp cocoa (unsweetened chocolate) powder
60 ml/4 tbsp boiling water
175 g/6 oz/¾ cup butter or margarine, at kitchen temperature
175 g/6 oz/¾ cup dark soft brown sugar
5 ml/1 tsp vanilla essence (extract)
3 eggs, at kitchen temperature
175 g/6 oz/1½ cups self-raising (self-rising) flour
15 ml/1 tbsp black treacle (molasses)
Butter Cream Icing
Icing (confectioners') sugar, for dusting (optional)

Closely line the base and sides of an 18 x 9 cm/7 x 3½ in diameter soufflé dish with clingfilm (plastic wrap), allowing it to hang slightly over the edge. Mix the cocoa smoothly with the boiling water. Cream together the butter or margarine, sugar and vanilla essence until light and fluffy. Beat in the eggs one at a time, adding 15 ml/1 tbsp flour with each one. Fold in the remaining flour with the black treacle until evenly combined. Spread smoothly into the prepared dish and cover loosely with kitchen paper. Cook on Full for 6–6½ minutes until the cake is well risen and no longer damp- looking on top. Do not overcook or the cake will shrink and toughen. Allow to stand for 5 minutes, then ease the cake out of its dish by holding the clingfilm (plastic wrap) and transfer to a wire rack. Gently peel away the wrap and leave to cool. Cut the cake horizontally into three layers and sandwich together with the icing (frosting). Dust the top with sifted icing sugar before cutting, if liked.

Chocolate Mocha Cake

Serves 8–10

Prepare as for Chocolate Butter Cream Layer Cake, but flavour the Butter Cream Icing (frosting) with 15 ml/1 tbsp very strong black coffee. For a more intense flavour, add 5 ml/1 tsp ground coffee with the liquid coffee.

Orange-choc Layer Cake

Serves 8–10

Prepare as for Chocolate Butter Cream Layer Cake, but add 10 ml/2 tsp finely grated orange peel to the cake ingredients.

Double Chocolate Cake

Serves 8–10

Prepare as for Chocolate Butter Cream Layer Cake, but add 100 g/4 oz/1 cup melted and cooled plain (semi-sweet) chocolate to the Butter Cream Icing (frosting). Allow to firm up before using.

Whipped Cream and Walnut Torte

Serves 8–10

1 Chocolate Butter Cream Layer Cake
300 ml/½ pt/1¼ cups double (heavy) cream
150 ml/¼ pt/2/3 cup whipping cream
45 ml/3 tbsp icing (confectioners') sugar, sifted
Any flavouring essence (extract), such as vanilla, rose, coffee, lemon, orange, almond, ratafia
Nuts, chocolate shavings, silver dragees, crystallised flower petals or glacé (candied) fruits, to decorate

Cut the cake horizontally into three layers. Beat together the creams until thick. Fold in the icing sugar and flavouring to taste. Sandwich the cake layers together with the cream and decorate the top as wished.

Christmas Gâteau

Serves 8–10

1 Chocolate Butter Cream Layer Cake
45 ml/3 tbsp seedless raspberry jam (conserve)
Marzipan (almond paste)
300 ml/½ pt/1¼ cups double (heavy) cream
150 ml/¼ pt/2/3 cup whipping cream
60 ml/4 tbsp caster (superfine) sugar
Glacé (candied) cherries and edible holly sprigs, to decorate

Cut the cake into three layers and sandwich together with the jam topped with thinly rolled out rounds of marzipan. Beat together the creams and caster sugar until thick and use to cover the top and sides of the cake. Decorate the top with cherries and holly.

American Brownies

Makes 12

50 g/2 oz/½ cup plain (semi-sweet) chocolate, broken into pieces
75 g/3 oz/2/3 cup butter or margarine
175 g/6 oz/¾ cup dark soft brown sugar
2 eggs, at kitchen temperature, beaten
150 g/5 oz/1¼ cups plain (all-purpose) flour
1.5 ml/¼ tsp baking powder
5 ml/1 tsp vanilla essence (extract)
30 ml/2 tbsp cold milk
Icing (confectioners') sugar, for dusting

Butter and base line a 25 x 16 3 5 cm/10 x 6½ 3 2 in dish. Melt the chocolate and butter or margarine on Full for 2 minutes, stirring until well mixed. Beat in the sugar and eggs until well combined. Sift together the flour and baking powder, then lightly stir into the chocolate mixture with the vanilla essence and milk. Spread evenly into the prepared dish and cover loosely with kitchen paper. Cook on Full for 7 minutes until the cake is well risen and the top is peppered with small broken air holes. Allow to cool in the dish for 10 minutes. Cut into squares, dust the tops fairly thickly with icing sugar, then leave to cool completely on a wire rack. Store in an airtight container.

Chocolate Nut Brownies

Makes 12

Prepare as for American Brownies, but add 90 ml/6 tbsp coarsely chopped walnuts with the sugar. Cook for 1 minute extra.

Oaten Toffee Triangles

Makes 8

125 g/4 oz/½ cup butter or margarine
50 g/2 oz/3 tbsp golden (light corn) syrup
25 ml/1½ tbsp black treacle (molasses)
100 g/4 oz/½ cup dark soft brown sugar
225 g/8 oz/2 cups porridge oats

Thoroughly grease a deep 20 cm/8 in diameter dish. Melt together the butter, syrup, treacle and sugar, uncovered, on Defrost for 5 minutes. Stir in the oats and spread the mixture into the dish. Cook, uncovered, on Full for 4 minutes, turning the dish once. Allow to stand for 3 minutes. Cook for a further 1½ minutes. Allow to cool to lukewarm, then cut into eight triangles. Remove from the dish when cold and store in an airtight container.

Muesli Triangles

Makes 8

Prepare as for Oaten Toffee Triangles, but substitute unsweetened muesli for the porridge oats.

Chocolate Queenies

Makes 12

125 g/4 oz/1 cup self-raising (self-rising) flour
30 ml/2 tbsp cocoa (unsweetened chocolate) powder
50 g/2 oz/¼ cup butter or margarine, at kitchen temperature
50 g/2 oz/¼ cup light soft brown sugar
1 egg
5 ml/1 tsp vanilla essence (extract)
30 ml/2 tbsp cold milk
Icing (confectioners') sugar or chocolate spread, to decorate (optional)

Sift together the flour and cocoa. In a separate bowl, cream together the butter or margarine and sugar until soft and fluffy. Beat in the egg and vanilla essence. Fold in the flour mixture alternately with the milk, stirring briskly with a fork without beating. Divide between 12 paper cake cases (cupcake papers). Place six at a time on the glass or plastic turntable, cover loosely with kitchen paper and cook on Full for 2 minutes. Cool on a wire rack. Dust with sifted icing sugar or cover with chocolate spread, if wished. Store in an airtight container.

Flaky Chocolate Queenies

Makes 12

Prepare as for Chocolate Queenies, but crush a small chocolate flake bar and gently stir it into the cake mixture after the egg and vanilla essence have been added.

Breakfast Bran and Pineapple Cake

Makes about 12 pieces

A fairly dense cake and a useful snack breakfast served with yoghurt and a drink.

100 g/3½ oz/1 cup All Bran cereal

50 g/2 oz/¼ cup dark soft brown sugar

175 g/6 oz canned crushed pineapple

20 ml/4 tsp thick honey

1 egg, beaten

300 ml/½ pt/1¼ cups skimmed milk

150 g/5 oz/1¼ cups self-raising (self-rising) wholemeal flour

Closely line the base and sides of an 18 cm/7 in diameter soufflé dish with clingfilm (plastic wrap), allowing it to hang very slightly over the edge. Put the cereal, sugar, pineapple and honey into a bowl. Cover with a plate and warm on Defrost for 5 minutes. Mix in the remaining ingredients, stirring briskly without beating. Transfer to the prepared dish. Cover loosely with kitchen paper and cook on Defrost for 20 minutes, turning the dish four times. Leave until cooled to just warm, then transfer to a wire rack by holding the clingfilm. When completely cold, store in an airtight container for 1 day before cutting.

Fruited Chocolate Biscuit Crunch Cake

Makes 10–12

200 g/7 oz/scant 1 cup plain (semi-sweet) chocolate, broken into squares

225 g/8 oz/1 cup unsalted (sweet) butter (not margarine)

2 large eggs, at kitchen temperature, beaten

5 ml/1 tsp vanilla essence (extract)

75 g/3 oz/¾ cup coarsely chopped mixed nuts

75 g/3 oz/¾ cup chopped crystallised pineapple or papaya

75 g/3 oz/¾ cup chopped crystallised ginger

25 ml/1½ tbsp icing (confectioners') sugar, sifted

15 ml/1 tbsp fruit liqueur, such as Grand Marnier or Cointreau

225 g/8 oz plain sweet biscuits (cookies) such as digestives (Graham crackers), each snapped into 8 pieces

Closely line the base and sides of a 20 cm/8 in diameter dish or sponge sandwich tin (pan) with clingfilm (plastic wrap). Melt the chocolate pieces in a large bowl, uncovered, on Defrost for 4–5 minutes until very soft but still holding their original shape. Cut the butter into large cubes and melt, uncovered, on Defrost for 2–3 minutes. Stir thoroughly into the melted chocolate with the eggs and vanilla essence. Mix in all the remaining ingredients. When well combined, spread into the prepared tin and cover with foil or clingfilm (plastic wrap). Chill for 24 hours, then carefully lift out and peel away the clingfilm. Cut into wedges to serve. Keep refrigerated between servings as the cake softens at room temperature.

Fruited Mocha Biscuit Crunch Cake

Makes 10–12

Prepare as for Fruited Chocolate Biscuit Crunch Cake, but melt 20 ml/4 tsp instant coffee powder or granules with the chocolate and substitute coffee liqueur for the fruit liqueur.

Fruited Rum and Raisin Biscuit Crunch Cake

Makes 10–12

Prepare as for Fruited Chocolate Biscuit Crunch Cake, but substitute 100 g/3½ oz/¾ cup raisins for the crystallised fruit and substitute dark rum for the liqueur.

Fruited Whisky and Orange Biscuit Crunch Cake

Makes 10–12

Prepare as for Fruited Chocolate Biscuit Crunch Cake, but stir the finely grated peel of 1 orange into the chocolate and butter and substitute whisky for the liqueur.

White Chocolate Fruited Crunch Cake

Makes 10–12

Prepare as for Fruited Chocolate Biscuit Crunch Cake, but substitute white chocolate for dark.

Two-layer Apricot and Raspberry Cheesecake

Serves 12

For the base:

100 g/3½ oz/½ cup butter

225 g/8 oz/2 cups chocolate digestive biscuit (Graham cracker) crumbs

5 ml/1 tsp mixed (apple-pie) spice

For the apricot layer:

60 ml/4 tbsp cold water

30 ml/2 tbsp powdered gelatine

500 g/1 lb 2 oz/2¼ cups curd (smooth cottage) cheese

250 g/9 oz/1¼ cups fromage frais or quark

60 ml/4 tbsp smooth apricot jam (conserve)

75 g/3 oz/2/3 cup caster (superfine) sugar

3 eggs, separated

A pinch of salt

For the raspberry layer:

45 ml/3 tbsp cold water

15 ml/1 tbsp powdered gelatine

225 g/8 oz fresh raspberries, crushed and sieved (strained)

30 ml/2 tbsp caster (superfine) sugar

150 ml/¼ pt/2/3 cup double (heavy) cream

For decoration:

Fresh raspberries, strawberries and strings of redcurrants

To make the base, melt the butter, uncovered, on Defrost for 3–3½ minutes. Stir in the biscuit crumbs and mixed spice. Spread evenly over the base of a 25 cm/10 in diameter springform cake tin (pan). Chill for 30 minutes until firm.

To make the apricot layer, put the water and gelatine into a basin and stir well to mix. Stand for 5 minutes until softened. Melt, uncovered, on Defrost for 2½–3 minutes. Put in a food processor with the curd cheese, fromage frais or quark, jam, sugar and egg yolks and run the machine until the ingredients are thoroughly combined. Scrape out into a large bowl, cover with a plate and chill until just beginning to thicken and set round the edge. Whisk the egg whites and salt to stiff peaks. Beat one-third into the cheese mixture, then fold in the remainder with a metal spoon or spatula. Spread evenly over the biscuit base. Cover loosely with kitchen paper and chill for at least 1 hour until firm.

To make the raspberry layer, put the water and gelatine into a basin and stir well to mix. Stand for 5 minutes until softened. Melt, uncovered, on Defrost for 1½–2 minutes. Combine with the raspberry purée and sugar. Cover with foil or clingfilm (plastic wrap) and chill until just beginning to thicken and set round the edge. Beat the cream until softly thickened. Beat one-third into the fruit mixture, then fold in the remainder with a metal spoon or spatula. Spread evenly over the cheesecake mixture. Cover loosely and chill for several hours until firm. To serve, run a knife dipped in hot water round the inside edge to loosen the cheesecake. Unclip the tin and remove the side. Decorate the top with fruits. Cut into portions with a knife dipped in hot water.

Peanut Butter Cheesecake

Serves 10

For the base:

100 g/3½ oz/½ cup butter

225 g/8 oz/2 cups ginger biscuit (cookie) crumbs

For the topping:

90 ml/6 tbsp cold water

45 ml/3 tbsp powdered gelatine

750 g/1½ lb/3 cups curd (smooth cottage) cheese

4 eggs, separated

5 ml/1 tsp vanilla essence (extract)

150 g/5 oz/2/3 cup caster (superfine) sugar

A pinch of salt

150 ml/¼ pt/2/3 cup double (heavy) cream

60 ml/4 tbsp smooth peanut butter, at kitchen temperature

Chopped lightly salted or plain peanuts (optional)

To make the base, melt the butter, uncovered, on Defrost for 3–3½ minutes. Stir in the biscuit crumbs. Spread over the base of a 20 cm/8 in diameter springform tin (pan) and chill for 20–30 minutes until firm.

To make the topping, put the water and gelatine into a basin and stir well to mix. Stand for 5 minutes to soften. Melt, uncovered, on Defrost for 3–3½ minutes. Put in a food processor with the cheese, egg yolks, vanilla essence and sugar and run the machine until smooth. Scrape out into a large bowl. Whisk the egg whites and salt to stiff peaks. Whip the cream until softly thickened. Fold the egg whites and cream alternately into the cheese mixture. Finally, swirl in the peanut butter. Spread evenly into the prepared tin, cover securely and chill for at least 12 hours. To serve, run a knife dipped in hot water round the side to loosen. Unclip the tin and remove the sides. Decorate with chopped peanuts, if liked. Cut into portions with a knife dipped in hot water.

Lemon Curd Cheesecake

Serves 10

Prepare as for Peanut Butter Cheesecake, but substitute lemon curd for the peanut butter.

Chocolate Cheesecake

Serves 10

Prepare as for Peanut Butter Cheesecake, but substitute chocolate spread for the peanut butter.

Sharon Fruit Cheesecake

Serves 10

A recipe, sent to me by a New Zealand lady, based on the tomato-like fruit tamarillo. As they are not always easy to obtain, winter sharon fruit make an admirable substitute, or even the look-alike persimmon as long as they are very ripe.

For the base:
175 g/6 oz/¾ cup butter
100 g/3½ oz/½ cup light soft brown sugar
225 g/8 oz malt biscuit (cookie) crumbs

For the filling:
4 sharon fruit, chopped
100 g/4 oz/½ cup light soft brown sugar
30 ml/2 tbsp powdered gelatine
30 ml/2 tbsp cold water
300 g/10 oz/1¼ cups cream cheese
3 large eggs, separated
Juice of ½ lemon

Thoroughly rinse a 25 cm/10 in diameter springform tin (pan) and leave wet. Melt the butter or margarine, uncovered, on Defrost for 3–3½ minutes. Stir in the sugar and biscuit crumbs. Press evenly over the base of the tin. Chill while preparing the cake filling.

To make the filling, put the sharon fruit into a dish and sprinkle with half the sugar. Put the gelatine into a basin and stir in the water. Stand for 5 minutes until softened. Melt, uncovered, on Defrost for 3–3½ minutes. In separate bowl, beat the cheese until soft and fluffy, then work in the gelatine, egg yolks, lemon juice and remaining sugar. Whisk the egg whites to stiff peaks. Fold into the cheese mixture alternatively with the sharon fruit. Spoon over the biscuit base and chill overnight. To serve, run a knife dipped in hot water round the side to loosen, then unclip the tin and remove the sides.

Blueberry Cheesecake

Serves 10

Prepare as for Sharon Fruit Cheesecake, but substitute 350 g/12 oz blueberries for the sharon fruit.

Baked Lemon Cheesecake

Serves 10

For the base:

75 g/3 oz/1/3 cup butter, at kitchen temperature
175 g/6 oz/1½ cups digestive biscuit (Graham cracker) crumbs
30 ml/2 tbsp caster (superfine) sugar

For the filling:

450 g/1 lb/2 cups medium-fat curd (smooth cottage) cheese, at kitchen temperature
75 g/3 oz/1/3 cup caster (superfine) sugar
2 large eggs, at kitchen temperature
5 ml/1 tsp vanilla essence (extract)
15 ml/1 tbsp cornflour (cornstarch)
Finely grated peel and juice of 1 lemon
150 ml/¼ pt/2/3 cup double (heavy) cream
150 ml/5 oz/2/3 cup soured (dairy sour) cream

To make the base, melt the butter, uncovered, on Defrost for 2–2½ minutes. Stir in the biscuit crumbs and sugar. Line the base and side of a 20 cm/8 in diameter dish with clingfilm (plastic wrap), allowing it to hang very slightly over the edge. Cover the base and sides with the biscuit mixture. Cook, uncovered, on Full for 2½ minutes.

To make the filling, beat the cheese until soft, then blend in the remaining ingredients except the soured cream. Pour into the crumb case and cover loosely with kitchen paper. Cook on Full for 12 minutes, turning the dish twice. The cake is ready when there is some movement to be seen in the middle and the top has risen slightly and is just beginning to crack. Allow to stand for 5 minutes. Remove from the microwave and gently spread with the soured cream, which will set on top and even out as the cake cools.

Baked Lime Cheesecake

Serves 10

Prepare as for Baked Lemon Cheesecake, but substitute the peel and juice of 1 lime for the lemon.

Baked Blackcurrant Cheesecake

Serves 10

Prepare as for Baked Lemon Cheesecake, but when completely cold spread the top with either good-quality blackcurrant jam (conserve) or canned blackcurrant fruit filling.

Baked Raspberry Cheesecake

Serves 10

Prepare as for Baked Lemon Cheesecake, but substitute raspberry blancmange powder for the cornflour (cornstarch). Decorate the top with fresh raspberries.

Beef and Pickled Onion

1 croissant

Creamed horseradish

2–3 slices cold roast beef

1 brown pickled onion, thinly sliced

Halve the croissant and spread the cut sides with creamed horseradish. Sandwich together with the beef and onion slices. Put on a plate and heat, uncovered, on Defrost for 30–35 seconds until warm.

Pizza Croissant

1 croissant

15–20 ml/3–4 tsp pesto

3 thin slices Mozzarella cheese

1 small tomato, thinly sliced

2 stoned (pitted) black olives (optional)

Halve the croissant and spread the cut sides with pesto. Sandwich together with the remaining ingredients. Put on a plate and heat, uncovered, on Defrost for 40 seconds until warm.

Cottage Cheese and Lemon

1 croissant

Lemon Curd

30 ml/2 tbsp cottage cheese

1 small apple, grated

Halve the croissant and spread the cut sides with lemon curd. Sandwich together with the cottage cheese and apple. Put on a plate and heat, uncovered, on Defrost for 25–30 seconds until warm.

Spicy Jam and Banana

1 croissant

15 ml/1 tbsp red jam (conserve)

1 small banana, sliced

Ground cinnamon

Halve the croissant and spread the cut sides with jam. Sandwich together with the banana slices and sprinkle with cinnamon. Put on a plate and heat, uncovered, on Defrost for 25–30 seconds until warm.

Chocolate and Banana

Prepare as for Spicy Jam and Banana, but substitute chocolate spread for the jam (conserve).

Baked Beans on Toast

A traditional favourite, microwaved on Defrost to prevent the beans bursting.

1 large slice toast
Butter or margarine (optional)
150 g/5 oz/2/3 cup baked beans in tomato sauce

Put the toast on a plate. Leave plain or spread with butter or margarine. Top with the beans. Heat, uncovered, on Defrost for 3½ minutes until warm.

Cheesy Beans on Toast

Serves 1

Prepare as for Baked Beans on Toast, but sprinkle 45 ml/3 tbsp grated Cheddar cheese on top of the beans. Cook for an extra 15–20 seconds.

Spaghetti on Toast

Serves 1

1 large slice toast
Butter or margarine (optional)
213 g/7½ oz/1 small can spaghetti in tomato sauce

Put the toast on a plate. Leave plain or spread with butter or margarine. Top with the spaghetti. Heat, uncovered, on Full for 2–2¼ minutes until warm.

Tipsy Trout

1 whole trout, cleaned and washed
15 ml/1 tbsp butter or margarine
Salt and freshly ground black pepper
Paprika
30 ml/2 tbsp sherry

Put the trout on a plate. Melt the butter or margarine, uncovered, on Full for 30 seconds. Stir in all the remaining ingredients and spoon over the fish. Cover with clingfilm (plastic wrap) and slit it twice to allow steam to escape. Cook on Defrost for 8 minutes. Allow to stand for 1 minute before eating.

Tuna Rarebit with Mayonnaise

1 large slice white or brown toast
30 ml/2 tbsp mayonnaise
100 g/3½ oz canned tuna in oil, flaked
30 ml/2 tbsp grated Cheddar cheese
Paprika

Put the toast on a plate and spread with the mayonnaise. Top evenly with the tuna. Sprinkle with the cheese and dust with paprika. Heat through, uncovered, on Full for 2 minutes.

www.ingramcontent.com/pod-product-compliance
Lightning Source LLC
Chambersburg PA
CBHW071818080526
44589CB00012B/840